1200 MCQs in Medicine

1200 MCQs
in Medicine

Michael J. Ford MBChB (Hons) MD FRCPE

Consultant Physician,
Eastern General Hospital, Edinburgh
Honorary Senior Lecturer in Medicine,
Edinburgh University, Edinburgh, UK

SECOND EDITION

CHURCHILL LIVINGSTONE
EDINBURGH LONDON MELBOURNE NEW YORK AND TOKYO 1991

CHURCHILL LIVINGSTONE
Medical Division of Pearson Professional Ltd

Distribution in the United States of America by
Churchill Livingstone Inc., 650 Avenue of the Americas,
New York, N.Y. 10011, and by associated companies,
branches and representatives throughout the world.

© Longman Group UK Limited 1991

First edition 1980
Second edition 1991
    Reprinted 1993 (twice)
    Reprinted 1995

First edition by P. R. Fleming

ISBN 0-443-04252-7

British Library Cataloguing in Publication Data
1200 MCQs in medicine – 2nd ed.
    1. Man. Diseases. Questions & answers
    I. Ford, Michael J. (Michael Joseph) 1949–616

Library of Congress Cataloguing in Publication Data
Ford, Michael J.
    1200 MCQs in medicine. – 2nd ed./Michael J. Ford.
        p.   cm.
    Rev. ed. of: 1200 MCQs in
medicine/edited by P. R. Fleming. 1980.
    1. Internal medicine – Examinations, questions, etc.
2. Physical diagnosis – Examinations, questions, etc.
I. Title II. Title: One thousand two hundred
MCQs in medicine
    [DNLM: 1. Diagnosis – examination questions.
2. Medicine – examination questions.
WB 18 F711z]
RC58.F66 1991
616´.0076 – dc20   90–15156
DNLM/DLC   CIP
for Library of Congress

The
publisher's
policy is to use
**paper manufactured
from sustainable forests**

Produced by Longman Singapore Publishers (Pte) Ltd
Printed in Singapore

Introduction

The eleven years since first publication of *1200 MCQs in Medicine* have seen enormous changes in the field of medicine. The construction of MCQs has also progressed during this time and in consequence a complete revision of the text has become increasingly necessary. The original concept by Dr P. R. Fleming of a book of MCQs supplementing *Davidson's Principles and Practice of Medicine* and *Macleod's Clinical Examination* was sound, and over the years the book has proved to be a useful and valued method of self-assessment for medical undergraduates and postgraduates. The aim of the book remains like that of its predecessor to help students increase the efficiency with which they acquire the factual knowledge necessary for good medical practice.

Though the questions have been arranged to correspond with the chapters of *Davidson's Principles and Practice of Medicine* Sixteenth Edition, the corresponding sections of *Macleod's Clinical Examination* have been integrated into the appropriate chapters. In addition, the content of the questions has been designed so that the book should prove useful to students using other medical textbooks including the *Textbook of Medicine* edited by Souhami and Moxham and *Clinical Medicine* edited by Kumar and Clark.

THE PRINCIPLES AND TECHNIQUE

Multiple choice questions are widely used for examination purposes as a reliable and discriminatory test of factual knowledge. Lack of familiarity with the MCQ format may result in unexpected failure, though more usually failure is attributable to a lack of adequate reading and understanding of clinical medicine and the basic sciences. Familiarity with the technique of MCQ examinations is no substitute for the systematic study required in modern medicine.

1. Read each stem question and the five items carefully. The questions have been carefully worded to avoid ambiguity and have not been designed to trick the unwary.
2. Identify the items which you can answer with confidence and record the answer TRUE or FALSE as appropriate.
3. Identify those items to which you do not know the answers. Do not guess the answer if you know nothing about the subject matter. Record the answer DO NOT KNOW and move to the next item.
4. There will be items the answers to which you may feel you know but lack confidence. After due consideration, record your answer provided it is not a blind guess but results from informed and intuitive reasoning.
5. Concentrate on each stem and item in turn rather than passing quickly from question to question. It is easier to concentrate on the problem in hand rather than to juggle with several unrelated questions simultaneously.

HOW TO USE THIS BOOK

Only the TRUE answers to the questions are listed at the foot of each page. Students preparing themselves for examinations are recommended to read the appropriate chapters of the textbooks and then to assess themselves using the MCQ technique described.

Record your answers and your reasoning before checking the correct answer. Then return to the appropriate section of a medical textbook and identify the reasons behind any differences of fact. Alternatively, work with fellow students in small groups using methods similar to those of the game *Trivial Pursuits*.

Edinburgh 1991   M.J.F.

Contents

Genetic factors in disease

1
In man
A somatic cell nuclei contain 22 pairs of homologous autosomes
B gamete nuclei are haploid with a single X or a Y chromosome
C the X chromosome is smaller than the Y chromosome
D an F body in somatic nuclei represents a Y chromosome
E a Barr-body is a genetically inactive X chromosome

2
In chromosomal disorders
A aneuploidy is the addition or deletion of a chromosome
B deletions arise from the loss of a segment of a chromosome
C ring chromosomes(r) are usually manifest as additions
D isochromosomes consist of two short arms(p) or long arms(q)
E translocation is the exchange of segments between chromosomes

3
The karyotype of
A a man is usually identified using bone marrow cells
B a female with Down's syndrome is 46, XX, – 21
C a male with Klinefelter's syndrome is 47, XXY
D a female with Turner's syndrome is 45, X0
E a male with Cri du chat syndrome is 46, XY, 5p-

4
Which of the following conclusions can be deduced from the pedigree shown below?
A the proband was a female in whom the disease was present
B the proband's grandparents were consanguineous
C one of the proband's parents had died of the disease
D the proband was a monozygotic twin
E the disease is transmitted in an autosomal recessive pattern

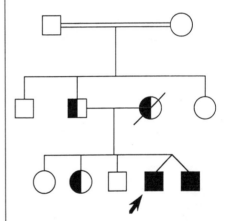

5
In the pedigree shown below
A the disease is transmitted by a dominant gene
B the proband's children will all be affected
C the patient A has a 50% chance of having affected children
D the pattern is typical of an X-linked dominant trait
E the inheritance pattern is compatible with an autosomal gene

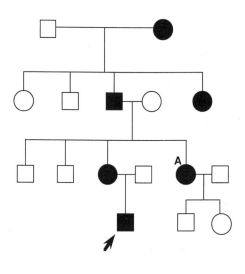

6
Given the marriage of two heterozygotes carrying the same gene transmitting an autosomal recessive disorder
A all of their healthy children will carry the gene
B there is a 10% chance that they are first cousins
C each of their children has a 1 in 4 chance of being affected
D 75% of families with an only child will have a healthy child
E 1 in 16 of their grandchildren will be affected

7
In a family affected by a disorder transmitted in an autosomal dominant mode
A non-penetrant genes could explain an unaffected generation
B the disorder invariably affects both sexes equally
C affected individuals are usually heterozygotes
D the disorder can occur without a previous family history
E 50% of the progeny of those affected are likely to be affected

8
In Down's syndrome
A due to trisomy-21 non-disjunction is the usual cause
B translocation accounts for 25% of those affected
C translocations often involve chromosomes 21 and 13, 14 or 15
D the majority of siblings have chromosomal abnormalities
E the commonest chromosomal abnormality is polyploidy

9
Characteristic features of Klinefelter's syndrome include
A Fallot's tetralogy
B mental retardation
C short stature
D sterility
E gynaecomastia

10
Characteristic features of Turner's syndrome include
A primary amenorrhoea
B tall stature
C webbing of the neck
D cubitus valgus
E aortic coarctation

Answers
5 A C D E
6 B C D

7 A C D E
8 A C
9 B D E
10 A C D E

11
Given a husband with haemophilia and his unaffected wife
A none of their sons will be affected
B all of their daughters will carry the haemophilic gene
C a daughter with Turner's syndrome will also have haemophilia
D all of his sisters will be carriers
E his maternal grandfather could have had haemophilia

12
The following disorders are transmitted in an autosomal dominant mode
A phenylketonuria
B polyposis coli
C achondroplasia
D cystic fibrosis
E Marfan's syndrome

13
The following disorders are transmitted in an X-linked recessive mode
A vitamin D resistant rickets
B Christmas disease
C nephrogenic diabetes insipidus
D haemochromatosis
E Duchenne muscular dystrophy

14
The following disorders are transmitted in an autosomal recessive mode
A albinism
B acute intermittent porphyria
C Friedrich's ataxia
D Wilson's disease
E Gilbert's syndrome

15
An X-linked dominant trait should be considered if
A both sexes are affected
B the family history reveals an excess of affected females
C the pedigree resembles that of an autosomal dominant trait
D all of the progeny of an affected female are affected
E half of the sons of an affected male are affected

16
The heritability of the first of the following pairs of diseases is greater than that of the second
A asthma — Huntington's chorea
B schizophrenia — Von Willebrand's disease
C ankylosing spondylitis – haemochromatosis
D type 1 diabetes mellitus — type II diabetes mellitus
E cleft lip — familial hypercholesterolaemia

17
The risk of a child developing congenital pyloric stenosis is greater if
A the child is female rather than male
B the mother rather than the father had the disorder
C two siblings rather than one sibling had the disorder
D the mother is aged 40 than if she is aged 20
E a brother was severely affected rather than mildly affected

18
Amniocentesis and/or chorionic villus biopsy are useful in establishing an antenatal diagnosis of
A Huntington's chorea
B Down's syndrome
C severe combined immunodeficiency
D anencephaly
E Duchenne muscular dystrophy

Answers
11 A B C E
12 B C E
13 B C E
14 A C E

15 A B C
16 D
17 B C E
18 B C D E

Immunological factors in disease

1
In the innate immune system
A neutrophil leucocytes phagocytose particulate antigens
B monocytes develop into tissue macrophages
C natural killer cells produce interferons
D acute phase proteins bind complement to enhance opsonisation
E macrophage-derived interleukin-1 mediates the febrile response

2
In the adaptive immune system
A small granular lymphocytes transform into killer cells
B T lymphocytes produce helper, suppressor and cytotoxic cells
C helper cells facilitate B cell-mediated killer cell activity
D delayed hypersensitivity reactions are mediated by T cells
E interleukin-2 is a lymphokine stimulating B cell proliferation

3
The following statements about immunoglobulins are true
A they are secreted by transformed T lymphocytes
B IgA is produced by B cells in the lamina propria of the gut
C IgG is the only immunoglobulin to cross the placental barrier
D IgA comprises 75% of the immunoglobulins in normal serum
E IgD is mainly found on the surface of B lymphocytes

4
The pathophysiological functions of immunoglobulins shown below are as follows
A IgG — neutralisation of soluble toxins
B IgA — agglutination of bacteria
C IgM — complement activation to produce cell lysis
D IgD — protection against viruses
E IgE — major regulator of B cell functions

5
The following statements about the complement system are true
A only the classical pathway produces both C3 and C5 convertases
B components of the classical pathway are mainly beta globulins
C the classical pathway is triggered by bacterial endotoxin
D the alternative pathway is triggered by immune complexes
E C1 esterase inhibitor deficiency produces angio-oedema

6
Mast cells
A are tissue eosinophils
B mediate delayed hypersensitivity
C can be activated by the complement components C3 and C5
D can be activated by opiate analgesics
E release leukotrienes, prostaglandins and histamine

Answers
1 A B C D E
2 B C D
3 B C E

4 A C
5 B E
6 C D E

7
In immediate (anaphylactic) hypersensitivity reactions
A eosinophils release histaminase to suppress inflammation
B the severity depends on the antigen's portal of entry
C eosinophils are attracted by basophil and mast cell products
D iv. adrenaline should be administered in systemic anaphylaxis
E urticaria often occurs in association with other features

8
In delayed hypersensitivity reactions
A T cells recruit macrophages in the development of the response
B the provoking infectious agents are typically extracellular
C antigen within the macrophage persists undestroyed
D contact eczema is usually caused by haptens such as nickel
E Langerhans cells in the dermis present the antigen in eczema

9
The deposition of immune complexes
A produces a vasculitis within vessel walls
B in tissues depends upon their size and local haemodynamics
C produces an Arthus reaction in the skin 10 days after exposure
D in serum sickness results in tissue damage within 12–24 hours
E in extrinsic allergic alveolitis is caused by IgA antibodies

10
Aetiological factors in the development of the spectrum of autoimmune disorders include
A loss of suppressor T cell control of helper T cells
B immunological exposure to sequestrated antigens
C bacterial mimicry of tissue antigen producing a cross-reaction
D drug-induced immune complexes activating complement
E genetic variations in the major histocompatibility complex

11
The following statements about the major histocompatibility complex (MHC) in man are true
A it is the HLA gene cluster on the long arm of chromosome 6
B it encodes the five classes of HLA antigens
C class 1 antigens are on all nucleated cells and not platelets
D class 2 antigens are on lymphocytes, monocytes and macrophages
E class 3 antigens consist of complement proteins

12
The following diseases are strongly associated with the HLA antigens shown below
A narcolepsy — DR2
B ankylosing spondylitis — B27
C myasthenia gravis — B8
D rheumatoid arthritis — A3
E haemochromatosis — DR4

Answers
7 A B C
8 A C D
9 A B

10 A B C D E
11 D E
12 A B C

13
The following statements about drugs and their effects on the immune system are true
A chlorpheniramine blocks all histamine receptors
B sodium cromoglycate inhibits the degranulation of mast cells
C adrenaline blocks the T cell release of lymphokines
D corticosteroids inhibit neutrophil adherence to endothelium
E cyclosporin suppresses B cells and T helper cells

14
In primary acquired hypogammaglobulinaemia
A there is an increased prevalence of autoimmune disease
B lymphocytes are usually present
C treatment with immunoglobulins each month is effective
D IgA deficiency is associated with gluten enteropathy
E hepatic granulomas are often present

15
In primary thymic hypoplasia (DiGeorge's syndrome)
A fungal and viral infections invariably occur
B serum immunoglobulin concentrations are normal
C there is severe lymphopenia
D thymic transplantation reverses the hypoparathyroidism
E neonatal death is usual

16
In acquired immunodeficiency syndrome (AIDS)
A the infectious agent is a retrovirus containing DNA
B the virus infects helper T lymphoctes
C B lymphocytes are activated to produce hypergammaglobulinaemia
D monocytes with the T4 surface antigen are also infected
E immune-mediated thrombocytopenia is common

Nutritional factors in disease

1
The daily essential nutrient requirements in man include
A 1–2 mg Vitamins D, K, and B_{12}
B 1–2 mg Vitamins A, B_1, B_6 and copper
C 50 g protein
D 50 mg Vitamin C
E 100 mg calcium and phosphate

2
The following statements about adult dietary energy resources are true
A carbohydrates yield 4 kcal/g
B fats yield 7 kcal/g
C sucrose, lactose and maltose are monosaccharides
D linoleic and linolenic acids are essential fatty acids
E proteins provide 4 kcal/g and all eight essential amino acids

3
A healthy daily diet for a slim, active man should comprise
A 1800 kcal (8.4 MJ)
B 50 g of carbohydrate
C 15 mg of both iron and zinc
D 60 g of protein of good biological value
E 20 μg of folic acid

4
The following statements about the basal metabolic rate (BMR) and energy balance in humans are true
A the BMR is the largest single component of energy expenditure
B the BMR increases with lean body mass and age
C the BMR is greater in females than males
D children require 2500 kcal per day
E the normal range of the body mass index (BMI) is 20–25 and is derived from the formula Weight(kg)/Height(m)^2

5
Clinical features of severe undernutrition in adults include
A a body mass index of 20–25
B oedema in the absence of hypoproteinaemia
C nocturia, cold intolerance and diarrhoea
D skin depigmentation, hair loss and covert infection
E cerebral atrophy and sinus tachycardia

6
Expected laboratory findings in severe undernutrition include
A decreased plasma free fatty acid concentrations
B increased plasma cortisol and reverse T_3 concentrations
C pancytopenia and impaired delayed skin sensitivity to tuberculin
D decreased plasma insulin, glucose and T_3 concentrations
E decreased urinary osmolality and creatinine excretion

Answers
1 B C D
2 A D E
3 C D

4 A D E
5 B C D
6 B C D E

7
The following statements about protein-energy malnutrition (PEM) are true
A kwashiorkor is a combined protein and calorie deficiency state
B nutritional marasmus occurs in pure dietary calorie deficiency
C dwarfism is usually associated with a body mass index of < 16
D there is an increased susceptibility to all types of infection
E premature weaning and childhood illnesses predispose to PEM

8
The clinical features of protein-energy malnutrition include
A marked muscle wasting and abdominal distension in marasmus
B weight loss more than growth retardation in marasmus
C hepatic steatosis and hypoproteinaemic oedema in kwashiorkor
D desquamative dermatosis, stomatitis and anorexia in marasmus
E associated zinc deficiency in kwashiorkor

9
The following statements about the treatment and prevention of severe protein-energy malnutrition are true
A mortality rates are around 20% even in hospitalised patients
B correction of fluid and electrolyte balance is vital
C restoration of calorie and protein intake can worsen the oedema
D fatty liver leads to cirrhosis if calorie intakes remain poor
E childhood mortality rates in developing countries could be halved by the adoption of breast feeding, oral rehydration, growth monitoring and immunisation.

10
The following statements about calcium balance in adult man are true
A total body calcium is about 1.2 kg of which 99% is in bone
B the UK recommended intake is 800 mg
C 50% of dietary calcium is excreted in the faeces
D dietary phytates and oxalates enhance calcium absorption
E one litre of cow's milk contains 600 mg of calcium

11
The following statements about iron balance in a healthy young adult female are true
A the healthy daily diet should provide 15 mg of iron
B 33% of dietary iron is absorbed
C organic iron (haem) is better absorbed than elemental iron
D daily iron losses of 1 mg results from desquamated cells
E 500 ml of blood contains 25 mg of iron

12
The following statements are true
A iodine deficiency produces goitre and thyrotoxicosis
B soft drinking water contains more fluoride than hard waters
C zinc deficiency produces dermatitis, hair loss and diarrhoea
D copper deficiency in children produces anaemia and poor growth
E phosphate deficiency occurs in neonates fed on cow's milk

13
Vitamin A
A is a fat-soluble vitamin
B is present as retinol in carrots and certain green vegetables
C deficiency results in xerophthalmia and keratomalacia
D daily intakes in adults of 10 mg are recommended
E is present is high concentrations in fish liver oils

Answers
  7 D E
  8 A B C E
  9 A B E

  10 A B
  11 A C
  12 C D
  13 A C E

14
Vitamin D
A is present in high concentrations in dairy products
B is non-essential in the diet given adequate sunlight exposure
C like vitamin A is stored mainly in the liver
D is converted to 1, 25 dihydroxycholecalciferol
E enhances calcium absorption by the induction of specific transport proteins in gut enterocytes

15
Rickets
A results from vitamin D deficiency before epiphyseal fusion
B in the UK occurs principally in the children of Asiatic origin
C is suggested by delayed motor milestones and dental eruption
D produces cranio-tabes and epiphyseal swelling of the ribs
E produces pectus excavatum and Harrison's sulci

16
Characteristic findings in severe rickets include
A epiphyseal expansion of the lower radius on X-ray
B hypophosphataemia due to secondary hyperparathyroidism
C hyperphosphaturia and an increased serum alkaline phosphatase
D deformities of the spine, pelvis and long bones
E undetectable concentrations of plasma 25-hydroxycholecalciferol

17
Characteristic findings in osteomalacia in adults include
A a significant reduction in total bone mass and bone osteoid
B presentation with persistent skeletal pain and bone tenderness
C proximal muscle weakness and a waddling gait
D rib, scapular and pelvic pseudo-fractures (Looser's zones)
E predisposing factors including partial gastrectomy, anti-convulsant therapy and renal impairment

18
Characteristic findings in generalised osteoporosis include
A chronic bone pain and impaired healing of bone fractures
B an association with alcohol abuse and malnutrition
C X-ray changes more marked in the limbs than the axial skeleton
D normal bone mineralisation but abnormal bone atrophy
E decreased serum calcium and phosphate concentrations

19
Vitamin K
A is a fat-soluble vitamin found in leafy vegetables
B is synthesised in the liver by the conversion of vitamin K_2
C is vital for the synthesis of clotting factors II, VII, IX and X
D deficiency in neonates results from the absence of normal gut flora
E absorption is inhibited by warfarin therapy

Answers
14 B D E
15 A B C D
16 A B C D E

17 B C D E
18 B D
19 A C D

20
Vitamin C (ascorbic acid) deficiency
A impairs wound healing due to defective collagen synthesis
B would develop within 4 months given a daily intake of 5 mg
C produces bleeding gums in edentulous individuals
D produces perifollicular haemorrhages and 'corkscrew' hairs
E in childhood produces anaemia and bone and joint pains

21
In thiamin (Vitamin B$_1$) deficiency
A anaerobic glycolysis is impaired resulting in lactic acidosis
B the diet is deficient in green vegetables and dairy products
C sudden death results from low output cardiac failure
D peripheral neuropathy results in marked muscle wasting
E Wernicke's encephalopathy is usually suggested by ataxia, confusion, nystagmus and conjugate gaze palsies

22
Deficiency of the following B vitamins is associated with the clinical syndromes listed below
A niacin — pellagra
B pyridoxine — isoniazid — induced peripheral neuropathy
C pantothenic acid — dermatitis, diarrhoea and dementia
D riboflavin — angular stomatitis and naso-labial seborrhoea
E biotin — hypercholesterolaemia and seborrhoeic dermatitis

23
The following statements about Vitamin B$_{12}$ and folic acid are true
A the serum B$_{12}$ is lower in strict vegetarians than meat-eaters
B both vitamins are essential for DNA synthesis
C a daily intake of 1–2 µg of vitamin B$_{12}$ is required
D a daily intake of 1–2 mg of folic acid is required
E deficiency of either vitamin produces a peripheral blood macrocytosis, pancytopenia and peripheral neuropathy

24
Which of the following vitamin deficiencies are suggested by the results of the biochemical assays shown below
A niacin — RBC transketolase
B pyridoxine — RBC glutamic oxaloacetic transaminase
C thiamin — RBC glutathione reductase
D tocopherol — RBC haemolysis with hydrogen peroxide
E riboflavin — RBC xanthurenic hydroxylase

25
The following statements about dietary fibre are true
A cereals increase stool bulk due to water-holding effects
B pulses increases stool bulk due to colonic bacterial growth
C pectins and gums retard gastric emptying
D colonic bacteria digest the polysaccharides to produce flatus
E average daily intakes of 15 g are inadequate

Answers
20 A B D E
21 C D E
22 A B D E

23 A B C E
24 B D
25 A B C D E

26
Patients with the following characteristics are at increased risk of malnutrition
A alcoholism
B major burns
C leukaemia receiving chemotherapy
D weight loss of 10% or more in the past 6 months
E body weight below 90% of standard for height

27
Characteristic findings in simple obesity in adults include
A a body mass index (BMI) > 30
B increased plasma cortisol, insulin and growth hormone levels
C a family history of obesity of similar degree and distribution
D onset in females at the menarche, in pregnancy or menopause
E basal metabolic rates, thermic responses to food and energy costs of exercise identical to those of lean subjects

28
Recognised associations of obesity include
A hyperuricaemia
B depression
C gallstones
D type II diabetes mellitus
E hyperlipoproteinaemia

29
Ideal weight reducing diets in the treatment of moderate obesity should
A provide no more than 500 kcal (2.1 MJ)
B theoretically achieve a weight loss of at least 2 kg per week
C be accompanied by anorectic drug therapy if weight loss ceases
D maintain nitrogen balance given a daily intake of 25 g protein
E reduce carbohydrate intake much more than total fat intake

Answers
26 A B C D
27 A C D E

28 A B C D E
29 none

Climate and the environment

1
The typical clinical features of sunburn include
A hypertension
B thirst and oliguria
C nausea and vomiting
D peripheral circulatory failure
E skin erythema and oedema is increased by aspirin-like drugs

2
The clinical features of heat syncope typically include
A headache
B postural hypotension
C fever
D warm dry skin
E nausea and vertigo

3
Prickly heat (miliaria rubra)
A affects negroes more often than caucasians
B arises from blocked sweat ducts within the prickle cell layer
C lesions occur predominantly on the exposed body areas
D is aggravated by air-conditioned rooms
E usually progresses to produce generalised erythroderma

4
The typical features of tropical anhidrotic asthenia include
A preexisting prickly heat
B insidious onset of headache and vertigo
C fever and hyperpyrexia
D thirst and oliguria
E peripheral cyanosis

5
In heat exhaustion
A water losses of 6–8 litres are typical
B headache, nausea and the absence of thirst are characteristic
C the skin is usually hot and dry
D progression to heatstroke is avoidable with effective therapy
E predominant water depletion is more common in the unacclimatised

6
Typical features of heat hyperpyrexia (heatstroke) include
A absence or impairment of sweat gland function
B body core temperature > 40 degrees C
C stigmata of salt and water depletion
D cold clammy skin with peripheral circulatory failure
E insidious onset progressing slowly to altered consciousness

7
Features consistent with a diagnosis of heatstroke include
A onset in a cool temperate climate
B history of exertion while wearing close-fitting garments
C development of acute renal failure
D coma and severe haemorrhage
E hypokalaemia and acute hepatic failure

8
Disorders predisposing to the development of hypothermia include
A Addison's disease
B hypothyroidism
C hepatic cirrhosis
D hypoglycaemia
E drug overdose

Answers
1 B C D
2 A B E
3 B
4 A B C

5 A B D
6 A B
7 A B C D E
8 A B C D E

9
The clinical features of hypothermia include
A hyponatraemia due to haemodilution
B body core temperature < 34 degrees C
C areflexia and absent pupillary responses
D ECG shows tachycardia with pronounced U waves
E asymptomatic acute pancreatitis and lactic acidaemia

10
The characteristic features of acute mountain sickness include
A onset at 1500 metres above sea level
B hyporeninaemia hypoaldosteronism
C headache, nausea and vomiting
D pulmonary and cerebral oedema
E hypocoagulation states

11
The typical features of chronic mountain sickness include
A alveolar hypoventilation
B inappropriate polycythaemia and chronic hypoxia
C relative protection from the disorder in sickle cell disease
D central cyanosis and cor pulmonale
E response to corticosteroid therapy

12
Diseases more common in tropical than temperate climates include
A chronic bronchitis
B bronchial asthma
C pericarditis
D colorectal carcinoma
E ischaemic heart disease

13
Liver disease in tropical Africa is particularly common due to
A cyanide in cassava
B ancylostomiasis
C trypanosomiasis
D hepatitis B infection
E aflatoxin in ground nuts

14
Environmental exposure to lead occurs
A principally from the inhalation of automobile emissions
B from the contamination of food and drink supplies
C in children from eating lead-based paint
D from lead water pipes and storage tanks
E normally in the UK resulting in blood lead levels = 1–3 mg/L

15
The features of chronic lead poisoning include
A inhibition of delta-aminolaevulinic acid dehydratase
B microcytic anaemia and punctate basophilia
C dysgeusia, constipation and abdominal pain
D gout and renal tubular acidosis
E peripheral neuropathy predominantly motor in type

16
Environmental exposure to mercury
A results mainly from the natural de-gassing of the earth's crust
B occurs as a result of the accumulation of mercury in sea fish
C is principally due to the use of mercury-containing fungicides
D in the smelting industry usually results in erethism
E was responsible for the epidemic of Minamata disease in Japan

---

Answers
 9 B C E
10 C D
11 A B D
12 C

13 C D E
14 B C D
15 A B C D E
16 A B E

17
The clinical features of chronic mercury poisoning include
A sensorineural deafness and constriction of the visual fields
B peripheral paraesthesiae and cerebellar ataxia
C erethism with sweating, flushing, excitability and memory loss
D acute pulmonary oedema, circulatory failure and renal failure
E intestinal mucosal necrosis with gastrointestinal bleeding

18
The clinical features of chronic fluorosis include
A more severe effects in adults than in children
B endemic occurrence in some tropical countries
C osteopetrosis and calcific enthesiopathy
D dental mottling and thickening of the long bones
E hypercalcaemia and renal calculi

19
Exposure to polychlorinated biphenyls (PCBs)
A occurs particularly commonly in sewage workers
B due to contaminated rice oil produces Yusho disease
C produces an acneiform rash and pigmentation
D causes watering eyes and an intractable cough
E causes foetal abnormalities and liver disease

20
The following statements about barotrauma in divers are true
A the greatest changes in barometric pressure occur below 10 metres
B shallow water blackout is due to hyperventilation and hypocarbia
C the lung volume doubles on ascending from 10 metres to the surface
D hyperinflation with air embolism occurs only in dives > 5 metres
E middle ear 'squeeze' typically ruptures the oval or round window

21
The following statements about decompression sickness are true
A symptoms are usually apparent within one hour of surfacing
B painful lymphoedema is typically due to thoracic duct obstruction
C dissolved nitrogen accumulates particularly in skeletal muscle
D headache, abdominal pain, vertigo and dyspnoea are characteristic
E recompression restores neurological normality even in subjects with paraplegia and hemiplegia

Answers
17 A B C
18 B C D
19 B C D E

20 B C
21 A D

Diseases due to infection

1
Diseases typically acquired from animals include
A leptospirosis
B bartonellosis
C Q fever
D Lyme disease
E hepatitis A

2
Diseases usually spread via the faecal-oral route include
A poliomyelitis
B cholera
C hepatitis E (non-A, non-B hepatitis)
D hepatitis B
E salmonellosis

3
Spread of the following infections is best prevented by
A use of insecticides in malaria
B active immunisation in measles
C barrier nursing in tuberculosis
D quarantine in diphtheria
E chemoprophylaxis in meningococcaemia

4
Schedules of immunisation in the UK should include
A BCG vaccination at the age of 5 years
B polio vaccine on 3 occasions during the first year of life
C mumps, measles and rubella at the age of 6 months
D diphtheria, tetanus and pertussis at 2, 3, and 4 months
E pre-school booster diphtheria, tetanus and polio vaccination

5
Contraindications to active immunisation include
A atopic disposition
B HIV infection if live vaccines are required
C pregnancy if live vaccines are required
D chronic cardiac or respiratory failure
E recent passive immunisation if live vaccines are required

6
Live viruses are usually used for active immunisation against
A poliomyelitis
B pertussis
C typhoid fever
D mumps, measles and rubella
E hepatitis B

7
Indications for passive immunisation with human immunoglobulin include
A hepatitis A and B
B tetanus
C rabies
D meningococcaemia
E syphilis

8
Notification is a statutory obligation in the following infections
A food poisoning
B leptospirosis
C viral hepatitis
D meningococcaemia
E measles and rubella

Answers
1 A C D
2 A B C E
3 A B D E
4 B D E

5 B C E
6 A D
7 A B C
8 A B C D E

9
Infections with an incubation period
< four weeks include
A chickenpox
B measles and rubella
C typhoid fever
D brucellosis
E tuberculosis

10
Infections with an incubation period
> four weeks include
A gonorrhoea
B meningococcaemia
C cholera
D schistosomiasis
E hepatitis B

11
Factors likely to be relevant in pyrexia of
unknown origin include
A travel abroad
B occupation
C leisure activities
D drug therapy
E animal contact

12
RNA viruses causing the following
infections include
A parvovirus — rubella-like syndrome
B reovirus — rotavirus gastroenteritis
C arenavirus — lymphocytic meningitis
D orthomyxovirus — influenza
E herpesvirus — chickenpox

13
DNA viruses causing the following
infections include
A adenovirus — acute tracheobronchitis
B cytomegalovirus — glandular fever-like
   illness
C togavirus — rubella
D picornavirus — hepatitis A
E rhinovirus — rabies

14
In the classification of HIV infection
A acute seroconversion simulating
   glandular fever = group I
B group II = persistent generalised
   lymphadenopathy
C group III = AIDS-related complex with
   constitutional disease
D group IV = includes thrombocytopenia
   and/or encephalitis-dementia
E asymptomatic infection = group II

15
Typical features of HIV infection at
presentation include
A hairy leucoplakia
B atypical pneumonia
C thrombocytopenic purpura
D pulmonary tuberculosis
E candidiasis and cryptosporidiosis

16
The development of AIDS due to HIV
infection is associated with
A RNA retrovirus infection
B depression of the suppressor rather than
   helper T lymphocytes
C encephalitis attributable to herpesvirus
   infection rather than HIV
D blindness which is usually attributable to
   cytomegalovirus retinitis
E Hodgkin's rather than non-Hodgkin's
   lymphoma

Answers
 9 A B C
10 D E
11 A B C D E
12 B C D

13 A B
14 A D E
15 A B C D E
16 A D

17
The typical features of measles include
A infection with a single-stranded RNA paramyxovirus
B rhinorrhoea and conjunctivitis at the onset
C Koplik's spots appear together with the skin rash
D the skin rash typically desquamates as it disappears
E infectivity is confined to the prodromal phase

18
Characteristic complications of measles include
A pneumonia
B post-viral encephalitis
C pancreatitis
D myocarditis
E otitis media

19
The typical features of rubella include
A infection with an RNA rhabdovirus spread by the faeco-oral route
B fever and polyarthralgia more marked in children than in adults
C infectivity for 7 days before and 4 days after the onset of the rash
D suboccipital lymphadenopathy with a macular rash behind the ears
E risk of serious foetal damage < 5% by the 16th week of pregnancy

20
Typical complications of rubella include
A 80% risk of foetal damage within the first 6 weeks of pregnancy
B post-viral encephalitis
C gastroenteritis and acute appendicitis
D polyarthritis
E pericarditis

21
The characteristic features of mumps include
A infection with an RNA paramyxovirus spread by the air-borne route
B high infectivity for 14–21 days after the onset of parotitis
C presentation with an acute lymphocytic meningitis
D abdominal pain which is usually attributable to mesenteric adenitis
E orchitis which is usually bilateral and predominantly occurs prepubertally

22
DNA herpes viruses produce the following infections
A roseola — herpes virus 6
B glandular fever — cytomegalovirus
C shingles — varicella-zoster virus
D interstitial pneumonitis — Epstein Barr virus
E bronchiolitis — respiratory syncytial virus

23
The clinical features of herpes simplex virus infections include
A recurrent labial or genital ulcers
B acute gingivostomatitis
C encephalitis
D shingles
E paronychia

24
The following statements about glandular fever are true
A infection is invariably attributable to the Epstein Barr virus
B presentation is usually with fever, headache and abdominal pain
C dysphagia and sore throat suggest CMV rather than EBV infection
D meningo-encephalitis and hepatitis are recognised complications
E severe oro-pharyngeal swelling requires prompt prednisolone therapy

Answers
17 A B D
18 A B E
19 C D E
20 A D

21 A C
22 A B C D
23 A B C E
24 B D E

25
The clinical features of chickenpox include

A infection due to varicella-zoster virus from air-borne spread

B high infectivity until 7 days after the last crop of vesicles

C useful response to acyclovir therapy in the immunocompromised

D palatal rash appears before involvement of the trunk then face

E constitutional symptoms are particularly severe in children

26
Recognised complications of chickenpox include

A pneumonia particularly in children rather than adults

B proliferative glomerulonephritis

C acute pancreatitis

D encephalitis with cerebellar involvement

E myocarditis

27
The characteristic features of rabies include

A rhabdovirus infection transmitted in animal saliva

B incubation period of 4–8 days

C the prognosis is invariably poor if symptoms develop

D encephalitis or ascending paralysis

E active and passive vaccination are useful in prevention and therapy

28
The clinical features of Lassa fever include

A fever, exudative pharyngitis and intercostal myalgia

B infection with an arenavirus transmitted in rats' urine

C renal, hepatic and circulatory failure

D incubation period of 2–3 months

E clinical response to tribavirin and immunoglobulin therapy

29
Features of Marburg and Ebola viral disease include

A arenavirus infection with an incubation period of 5–10 days

B fever, headache, myalgia and diarrhoea

C maculopapular rash and lymphadenopathy

D mucosal haemorrhages and pneumonia

E encephalitis and renal failure

30
The following statements about arboviruses are true

A they comprise togaviruses and bunyaviruses

B transmission is typically by the ingestion of infected water

C they occur predominantly in temperate climates

D the incubation period is usually more than 1 month

E complications include encephalitis and haemorrhage

31
The clinical features of yellow fever include

A a togavirus infection transmitted by mosquitoes

B an incubation period of 3–6 weeks

C peripheral blood leucocytosis in contrast to viral hepatitis

D fever, headache and severe myalgia with bone pains

E jaundice and renal failure due to haemolytic anaemia

Answers
25 A B C D
26 B D E
27 A C D E
28 A B C E

29 A B C D E
30 A E
31 A D E

32
Features of dengue (sandfly fever) include
A mosquito-borne infection with an incubation period of 3–6 days
B progression to acute circulatory, hepatic and renal failure
C rigors, headache, photophobia and backache are characteristic
D morbilliform rash and cervical lymphadenopathy
E protection by vaccination every 10 years in endemic areas

33
Diseases attributable to chlamydial infection include
A psittacosis
B Rift valley fever
C trachoma
D lymphogranuloma venereum
E Q fever

34
In trachoma
A blepharospasm is an invariable early feature
B upper eyelid follicular conjunctivitis is typical
C acute ophthalmia neonatorum is a recognised presentation
D tetracycline eye drops and oral sulphonamide therapy are indicated
E blindness is usually due to cataracts

35
The typical features of psittacosis include
A an incubation period of 2 weeks
B constitutional upset with fever, headache and myalgia
C pulmonary infiltrates on chest X-ray not apparent clinically
D birds surviving the disease are no longer infectious
E prompt resolution with sulphonamide therapy

36
Diseases attributable to mycoplasmal infection include
A haemolytic anaemia
B salpingitis
C pneumonia
D epididymoorchitis
E urethritis and prostatitis

37
Rickettsial infection is transmitted by
A infected water
B lice
C mosquitoes
D mites
E fleas

38
The typical clinical features of typhus fevers include
A rickettsial infection from arthropods
B parasitisation of the endothelium of small blood vessels
C fever, headache and backpain and cutaneous haemorrhages
D morbilliform rash, bronchopneumonia and splenomegaly
E response to chloramphenicol or tetracycline therapy

39
Clinical features consistent with the diagnosis of Q fever include
A exposure to sheep, cattle and unpasteurised milk
B an incubation period of 1–2 weeks
C pneumonia in the absence of fever, headache or myalgia
D blood culture-negative endocarditis
E prompt clinical response to sulphonamide therapy

Answers
32 A C D
33 A C D
34 B C D
35 A B C

36 A B C E
37 B D E
38 A B C D E
39 A B D

40
The clinical features of Lyme disease include
A infection with the tick-borne spirochaete Borrelia burgdorferi
B an expanding erythematous rash (erythema chronicum migrans)
C fever with headache, meningism and migratory musculoskeletal pains
D asymmetrical large joint recurrent oligoarthritis
E response to tetracycline or penicillin therapy

41
The clinical features of relapsing fevers include
A infection with borrelial spirochaetes
B an incubation period of 1–3 months
C rigors, headache, mental confusion and jaundice
D hepatosplenomegaly and thrombocytopenic purpura
E response to erythromycin or tetracycline therapy

42
The typical features of leptospirosis include
A incubation period of 1–3 months
B exposure to abbatoirs, farms, and inland waterways
C fever, severe myalgia, headache and conjunctival suffusion
D meningitis suggests Leptospira icterohaemorrhagica rather than L. canicola
E myocarditis, hepatitis and acute renal failure

43
Sexually-transmissible viral diseases include
A cytomegalovirus
B hepatitis A, B and non-A, non-B
C papovavirus
D herpes simplex
E molluscum contagiosum

44
The following statements about syphilis are true
A infection is usually caused by Treponema pertenue
B untreated, infectivity is restricted to the first two months
C the subdivision between early and late syphilis is at two years
D the incubation period for primary syphilis is typically 2–4 weeks
E tertiary and quarternary syphilis usually develop within 5 years

45
The characteristic features of secondary syphilis include
A fever and a macular rash occurring 8 weeks after the chancre
B condylomata lata in the moist areas appearing as flat papules
C generalised lymphadenopathy and oro-genital mucous ulceration
D CSF pleocytosis in 90% indicating meningovascular involvement
E soft early diastolic murmur on cardiac auscultation

46
Typical features of late (tertiary and quaternary) syphilis include
A latent period of at least 10 years after the initial infection
B destructive granulomas (gummas) in bones, joints and the liver
C chronic basal meningitis with cranial neuropathies
D tabo-paresis and aneurysms of the ascending aorta
E poor response of gummas to antibiotic therapy

Answers
40 ABCDE
41 ACDE
42 BCE
43 ABCDE

44 CD
45 ABC
46 ABD

47
The typical clinical features of gonorrhoea include
A an incubation period of 2–3 weeks
B anterior urethritis and cervicitis
C right hypochondrial pain due to perihepatitis
D haemorrhagic pustular rash and acute large joint oligoarthritis
E good response to spectinomycin therapy in penicillin allergy

48
Features suggestive of non-gonococcal urethritis include
A urethral culture of *Chlamydia trachomatis*
B urethral culture of *Ureaplasma urealyticum*
C keratoderma and peripheral oligoarthritis
D painless genital ulceration
E good response to penicillin therapy

49
The typical features of lymphogranuloma venereum include
A Donovan bodies within mononuclear cells on histology of the lesion
B transient genital ulceration 1–5 weeks after chlamydial infection
C fever, weight loss and inguinal lymphadenopathy
D proctitis and anal fistulae
E response to tetracycline therapy

50
Chancroid is associated with the following clinical features
A infection due to Donovania granulomatis
B an incubation period of 2–8 weeks
C painful genital ulcerated papules and lymphadenopathy
D progression to salpingitis and epididymoorchitis
E prompt response to penicillin therapy

51
Granuloma inguinale is associated with
A infection with *Haemophilus ducreyi*
B ulcerating granulomatous genital papules
C urethral, anal and vaginal strictures
D polyarthritis, aortitis and uveitis
E prompt response to penicillin therapy

52
Anogenital herpes simplex is typically associated with
A type I rather than type II herpes simplex viral infection
B primary attacks more severe and prolonged than recurrent attacks
C fever with painful genital ulceration and lymphadenopathy
D sacral dermatomal pain and urinary retention
E absence of clinical response to oral acyclovir

53
Scarlet fever is typically associated with
A rigors, headache and acute pharyngitis or tonsillitis
B generalised punctate erythema desquamating on resolution
C group B rather than group A streptococcal infection
D generalised rather than localised lymphadenopathy
E punctate erythma involving the face more than the limbs

54
The typical features of erysipelas include
A group A haemolytic streptococcal skin infection
B absence of constitutional symptoms
C well-defined area of cutaneous erythema and oedema
D commoner in young rather than elderly patients
E prompt response within 48 hours to benzyl penicillin

Answers
47 B C D E
48 A B C
49 A B C D E
50 C

51 B C
52 B C D
53 A B
54 A C E

55
Staphylococcal infection is associated with
A resistance to benzyl penicillin therapy
B necrotising enterocolitis
C bronchopneumonia
D toxic shock syndrome
E cellulitis

56
The clinical features suggesting toxic shock syndrome include
A onset 24–48 hours after food ingestion
B fever, myalgia, vomiting and diarrhoea
C hypotension and hypovolaemia
D prompt clinical response to benzyl penicillin
E generalised erythema desquamating on resolution

57
In bacteraemic shock
A endotoxin initiates disseminated intravascular coagulation
B peripheral vascular resistance falls initially
C acute circulatory failure is usually due to cardiac failure
D leucocytosis and thrombocythaemia indicate a poor prognosis
E antibiotic therapy should await bacteriological results

58
Diphtheria rather than streptococcal tonsillitis is suggested by
A tender cervical lymphadenopathy
B blood-stained nasal discharge and marked tachycardia
C firm, adherent tonsillar exudate extending beyond the tonsils
D paralysis of the soft palate, accommodation or ocular muscles
E an incubation period of 2–4 days followed by marked fever

59
In the treatment of diphtheria
A antitoxin should be avoided pending bacteriological confirmation
B antitoxin-induced anaphylaxis is best treated with prednisolone
C antitoxin-induced serum sickness produces intense bronchospasm
D isolation is usually unnecessary
E myocarditis typically results in permanent cardiac impairment

60
In whooping cough
A the incubation period is 1–2 weeks
B onset with rhinitis and conjunctivitis is characteristic
C paroxysmal coughing bouts develop 2–3 weeks after exposure
D Bordetella pertussis is best obtained from anterior nasal swabs
E antibiotic therapy significantly reduces coughing bouts

61
The typical features of meningococcal infection include
A air-borne spread of infection
B abrupt onset with headache, vomiting and meningism
C acute circulatory failure and purpuric rash
D isolation of serogroups A and C more commonly than group B
E control of infection in contacts is best achieved by vaccination

62
Characteristic features of tetanus include
A an incubation period of 2–3 days
B local muscular spasm precedes the onset of trismus
C convulsions associated with loss of consciousness
D abdominal rigidity without pain or tenderness
E bacteriological isolation of Clostridium tetani from the wound

---

Answers
55 A B C D E
56 B C E
57 A B
58 B C D

59 none
60 A B C
61 A B C
62 B D

63
In the treatment of tetanus
A tetanus toxoid should be given intravenously as soon as possible
B wound debridement should be undertaken prior to any other therapy
C human antitetanus immunoglobulin should be given immediately
D diazepam should be avoided because of the hazards of oversedation
E penicillin or metronidazole therapy should be administered

64
The typical features of botulism include
A ingestion of infected water 2–4 hours prior to symptom onset
B onset with an afebrile gastroenteritis or postural hypotension
C autonomic neuropathy induced by the cholinergic neurotoxin
D ocular neuropathy and bulbar palsy developing over 3 days
E dramatic clinical response to parenteral antitoxin

65
Clinical features of anthrax include
A occupational exposure to animals and animal products
B an incubation period of 1–3 weeks
C a painless cutaneous papule with regional lymphadenopathy
D gastroenteritis, meningitis or bronchopneumonia
E multiple antibiotic resistance is common

66
Recognised features of brucellosis include
A an incubation period of 3 months
B fever, night sweats and backpain
C hepatosplenomegaly and epididymoorchitis
D oligoarthritis and spondylitis
E peripheral blood neutrophil leucocytosis

67
Typical clinical features of yersiniosis include
A infection associated with the ingestion of polluted water
B acute regional ileitis and mesenteric adenitis
C erythema nodosum and reactive arthritis
D aseptic meningitis
E prompt response to penicillin therapy

68
The characteristic features of plague include
A an incubation period of less than 7 days
B transmission of Yersinia pestis in infected fish
C presentation is predominantly pneumonic rather than bubonic
D rigors, severe headache and painful lymphadenopathy
E absence of splenomegaly or hepatomegaly

69
The typical features of typhoid fever include
A faecal-oral spread of *Salmonella typhi* by food handlers
B an incubation period of 3–7 days
C onset with fever, headache, myalgia and septicaemia
D 'rose spots' on the trunk and splenomegaly 7–10 days after onset
E diarrhoea and abdominal pain and tenderness 10–14 days after onset

70
Recognised complications of typhoid fever include
A cholecystitis
B meningitis
C endocarditis
D osteomyelitis
E pneumonia

Answers
63 C E
64 B C D
65 A C D
66 B C D

67 B C
68 A D
69 A C D E
70 A B C D E

71
Paratyphoid fever rather than typhoid fever is suggested by
A onset with vomiting and diarrhoea
B an incubation period of 5–7 days
C absence of an erythematous macular rash
D the development of a reactive arthritis
E prominence of intestinal complications

72
In the diagnosis of the enteric fevers
A positive blood cultures usually develop 10–14 days after onset
B positive stool cultures are likeliest within 7 days of onset
C peripheral blood neutrophil leucocytosis is typically marked
D the Widal reaction is usually diagnostic within 7 days of onset
E persistent fever despite antibiotics indicates resistant organisms

73
The following symptom patterns suggest specific food poisoning
A bloody diarrhoea after 12–48 hours — Campylobacter jejuni infection
B vomiting and abdominal pain after 3–6 hours — staphylococcal toxin
C vomiting and abdominal pain after 30–90 minutes — food allergy
D bloody diarrhoea after 24–48 hours — *Escherichia coli* infection
E vomiting and diarrhoea after 12–48 hours — salmonella infection

74
Bacillary dysentery in the UK
A is usually caused by Shigella dysenteriae
B has an incubation period of 1–7 days
C often arises from contaminated water supplies
D is characterised by profuse watery diarrhoea
E should be treated with sulphonamide or tetracycline therapy

75
The characteristic features of untreated cholera include
A the recent ingestion of contaminated water or shellfish
B an incubation period of 5–10 days
C sudden onset of profuse watery diarrhoea followed by vomiting
D acute circulatory failure developing within 12 hours of onset
E rapidly progressive metabolic alkalosis and dehydration

76
Bartonellosis
A is transmitted by cattle flies in West Africa
B has an incubation period of 14–21 days
C typically causes fever, haemolytic anaemia and myalgia
D is diagnosed by the presence of bacilli within erythrocytes
E causes cherry-red cutaneous nodules appearing after 4–6 weeks

77
The typical features of melioidosis include
A infection with Pseudomonas pseudomallei via skin abrasions
B fever, pneumonia and hepatosplenomegaly
C chest X-ray appearances simulating acute tuberculosis
D positive urine cultures during the second week of fever
E resistance to conventional antibiotic therapy

Answers
71 A B
72 none
73 A B C D E
74 B

75 A C D
76 B C D E
77 A B C

78
The following statements about penicillins are true
A all penicillins are bactericidal
B like the cephalosporins, they contain a beta-lactam ring
C clavulanic acid inhibitis bacterial beta-lactamase
D they can safely be used in cephalosporin-allergic patients
E they should be given intrathecally in bacterial meningitis

79
Tetracycline therapy
A is bactericidal to sensitive bacteria
B is contraindicated in pregnancy
C doxycycline can safely be used in renal failure
D in acne is effective due solely to its antibacterial actions
E is active against rickettsiae, mycoplasmas and chlamydiae

80
The aminoglycosides
A are all ototoxic and nephrotoxic
B should be avoided in patients requiring frusemide therapy
C have ototoxic effects which are age-related
D are effective against anaerobes and *Streptococcus faecalis*
E should be avoided in renal failure

81
Erythromycin is active against the following microorganisms
A *Campylobacter jejuni*
B *Escherichia coli*
C *Legionella pneumophila*
D *Mycoplasma pneumoniae*
E *Clostridium welchii*

82
Chloramphenicol is active against the following microorganisms
A *Haemophilus influenzae*
B *Salmonella typhi*
C *Klebsiella pneumoniae*
D *Pseudomonas aeruginosa*
E *Brucella abortus*

83
Cotrimoxazole is active against the following microorganisms
A *Escherichia coli*
B *Brucella abortus*
C *Proteus mirabilis*
D *Streptococcus pneumoniae*
E *Haemophilus influenzae*

84
The following statements about antibiotic therapy are true
A chloramphenicol therapy should be avoided in neonates
B metronidazole is effective in giardiasis and amoebiasis
C cotrimoxazole is effective in pneumonia due to pneumocystis
D sodium fusidate is effective in staphylococcal osteomyelitis
E erythromycin is effective in pertussis

85
Indications for appropriate chemoprophylaxis include
A erythromycin in diphtheria contacts
B rifampicin in meningococcal contacts
C penicillin following previous rheumatic fever
D isoniazid in susceptible TB contacts
E amoxycillin in cardiac valve disorders during dental surgery

---

Answers
78 A B C
79 B C E
80 A B C E
81 A C D

82 A B C
83 A B C D E
84 A B C D E
85 A B C D E

86
Antiviral agents active against the following viruses include
A ganciclovir — cytomegalovirus
B amantadine — orthomyxovirus
C tribavirin — respiratory syncytial virus
D zidovudine — retrovirus
E acyclovir — herpes simplex and zoster virus

87
Characteristic features of leprosy include
A an incubation period of 2–5 years
B growth of the organism on Lowenstein-Jensen medium over 2–3 months
C spread of the tuberculoid form on prolonged patient contact
D spontaneous healing of the earliest macule
E a cell-mediated immune response in the lepromatous form

88
Typical features of tuberculold leprosy include
A cell-mediated immune response around nerves and hair follicles
B absence of infectivity of affected patients
C palpable thickening of the peripheral nerves
D development of erythema nodosum leprosum
E persistently negative lepromin skin test

89
Typical features of lepromatous leprosy include
A absence of infectivity of affected patients
B unlike the tuberculoid form, organisms are scanty in number
C blood-borne spread from the dermis throughout the body
D strongly positive lepromin skin test
E anaesthetic hypopigmented skin macules and plaques

90
Type 1 lepra reactions
A occur predominantly in lepromatous forms of leprosy
B are precipitated by the introduction of chemotherapy
C produce a painful inflammation of skin and nerve lesions
D typically progress to caseation of skin and nerve lesions
E result in the rapid loss of nerve function

91
Type 2 lepra reactions
A occur particularly in lepromatous forms of leprosy
B are the result of immune-mediated vasculitis
C typically produce fever and erythema nodosum leprosum
D produce iritis, orchitis and nerve pain and tenderness
E usually develop in the second year of chemotherapy

92
The following features are typical of borderline leprosy
A in Asia, most patients have the borderline lepromatous form
B in Africa, most patients have the borderline tuberculoid form
C skin lesions are bizarre and the eyes and nose are spared
D nerve lesions are less numerous than in tuberculoid leprosy
E lepra reactions are rare unlike the more polar forms of leprosy

---

Answers
86 A B C D E
87 A D
88 A B C
89 C

90 B C E
91 A B C D E
92 A B C

93
In the treatment of multi-bacillary leprosy
A the combination of rifampicin, clofazimine and dapsone is advisable

B patients should be isolated for the first week of chemotherapy

C rifampicin should be given for two days every month

D clofazimine and dapsone should be administered daily

E treatment should be continued for two years

94
The following statements about the life cycle of plasmodia are true
A sporozoites disappear from the blood within minutes of innoculation

B merozoites re-entering RBCs undergo sexual or asexual development

C all plasmodia first multiply in the liver then subsequently in RBCs

D dormant hypnozoites remain within the liver cells in all species

E fertilisation of the gametocytes occurs in the human RBCs

95
All species of plasmodia producing malaria in humans
A are transmitted exclusively by anopheline mosquitoes

B have a persistent exo-erythrocytic phase often dormant for years

C produce the initial symptoms on the release of RBC sporozoites

D parasitise RBCs and normoblasts in all stages of development

E parasitise capillary endothelium throughout the body

96
Typical features of *Plasmodium falciparum* malaria include
A febrile response more marked than in other forms of malaria

B absence of intravascular haemolysis and splenomegaly

C infected RBCs cause capillary occlusion throughout the body

D paucity of infection in haemoglobin S or C heterozygotic subjects

E longer incubation period of 3–4 weeks in non-immune individuals

97
Recognised clinical features of malaria include
A absence of *P. vivax* in subjects lacking the Duffy blood group

B asymptomatic P. malariae parasitaemia persisting for years

C rarity of clinical relapses beyond two years

D presentation with rigors, herpes simplex and haemolytic anaemia

E flu-like symptoms, jaundice and hepatosplenomegaly in P. falciparum

98
Complications of *Plasmodium falciparum* malaria include
A delirium and coma

B blackwater fever

C acute renal failure

D acute liver failure

E acute cardiac failure

Answers
93 A B C D E
94 A B C
95 none

96 C D E
97 A B C D E
98 A B C D E

99
The typical features of tropical splenomegaly syndrome include
A peripheral blood and bone marrow plasmacytosis simulating myeloma
B occurrence in hyperendemic areas of malaria
C high serum antibody titres to malaria but low parasitaemia
D marked elevation of the serum IgG concentration
E excellent clinical response to splenectomy

100
Appropriate drug therapy in malaria includes
A chloroquine except in P. ovale and P. vivax infections
B intravenous quinine in serious infections with P. falciparum
C sulfadoxine alone for P. falciparum infections in Central Africa
D chloroquine for 3–7 days for non-P. falciparum infections
E pyrimethamine and dapsone once weekly for prophylaxis in S.E. Asia

101
The clinical features of amoebic dysentery typically include
A an incubation period of 7–10 days
B presentation with profuse watery diarrhoea
C colonic mucosal involvement most marked in the rectum
D characteristic appearances of the mucosa on sigmoidoscopy
E Ent.histolytica cysts in the stool are pathognomonic of disease

102
Recognised complications of amoebiasis include
A severe intestinal haemorrhage
B expectoration of amoebic pus from a liver abscess
C cerebral abscess
D amoebomas of the caecum, colon and rectum
E genital and perineal ulceration from cutaneous amoebiasis

103
In the diagnosis and therapy of amoebiasis
A amoebic liver abscesses usually reveal the presence of cysts
B stool trophozoites are unlikely in the presence of blood and mucus
C hepatic abscesses are best identified by liver ultrasound scanning
D metronidazole therapy is effective in both liver and colonic disease
E furamide therapy should also be given to eliminate colonic cysts

104
The characteristic features of giardiasis include
A an incubation period of 2–3 days
B infection transmitted by air-borne droplet spread
C predominant parasitisation of the duodenum and jejunum
D presentation with watery diarrhoea and malabsorption
E clinical response to metronidazole or tinidazole

105
The typical clinical features of cryptosporidiosis include
A acute onset of watery diarrhoea
B weight loss and persistent diarrhoea for 4–6 weeks
C history of animal or bird contact
D self-limiting disease resolving without therapy
E prompt response to spiramycin therapy

Answers
 99 B C
100 B D E
101 D

102 A B C D E
103 C D E
104 C D E
105 A D

106
Recognised features of toxoplasmosis include
A infection derived from cats, pigs and sheep
B asymptomatic infection is common in otherwise healthy subjects
C congenital infection produces chorioretinitis and cerebral palsy
D a glandular fever-like illness with peripheral blood monocytosis
E pyrimethamine and sulphadimidine therapy is useful in AIDS

107
The typical features of African trypanosomiasis include
A transmission of the parasite by the tsetse cattle fly
B an incubation period of 2–3 weeks
C onset with a chancre-like skin lesion with local lymphadenopathy
D generalised lymphadenopathy, hepatosplenomegaly and encephalitis
E good prognosis given prompt pentamidine or suramin therapy

108
The typical features of South American trypanosomiasis include
A spread of the parasite by the reduviid bug of cats and dogs
B Romana's sign with eye closure due to a conjunctival lesion
C a latent period of many years before the onset of chronic disease
D colonic, biliary and oesophageal dilatation due to a neuropathy
E response to nifurtimox therapy achieves cure rates of 90%

109
Typical features of visceral leishmaniasis (kala-azar) include
A spread of Leishmania donovani by sandflies from dogs and rodents
B an incubation period of 1–2 weeks
C rigors with hepatomegaly without splenomegaly or lymphadenopathy
D diagnosis confirmed on peripheral blood film and blood cultures
E clinical response to pentavalent antimonials e.g. stibogluconate

110
Typical features of South American leishmaniasis include
A nasal and mouth mucosal ulcers
B painful ulcers in the groins or axillae
C marked splenomegaly and lymphadenopathy
D chronic ulcers on the pinna of the ear
E negative Leishmanin skin test

111
All forms of schistosomiasis are associated with
A trematode helminths reproducing in freshwater snails
B the passage of cercariae in the urine and/or stool
C cercarial penetration of the skin or mucous membranes
D progression to portal or pulmonary hypertension
E eradication following praziquantel therapy

112
The typical features of *Schistosoma haematobium* infection include
A disease confined to the urinary tract
B presentation with painless haematuria
C spontaneous resolution within a year after leaving an endemic area
D involvement of the uterine cervix and seminal vesicles
E an endemic disease in China and the Far East

Answers
106 A B C D E
107 A B C D E
108 A B C D E

109 A E
110 A D
111 A C E
112 B D

113
The typical features of *Schistosoma mansoni* infection include
A an endemic disease in Egypt and East Africa
B abdominal pain with loose, blood-stained stools
C progression to jaundice and chronic liver failure
D paraplegia, cor pulmonale and bowel papillomata
E weight loss and malabsorption due to small bowel disease

114
The typical features of *Schistosoma japonicum* infection include
A parasitisation of rodents and domestic animals in addition to man
B infestation follows the ingestion of raw fish and crustacea
C abdominal pain and diarrhoea due to ileal and colonic involvement
D epilepsy, hemiplegia, paraplegia and blindness
E morbidity and mortality rate less than that from the other species

115
The typical clinical features of paragonimiasis include
A ingestion of raw crustacea infected by the freshwater snail
B presentation with recurrent haemoptyses and chest pain
C pulmonary, intraabdominal and hepatic abscesses
D encephalitis, myelitis, gastroenteritis and hepatitis
E resistance to praziquantel therapy

116
Typical features of fluke infestation of the biliary tree include
A parasitisation by clonorchis, opisthorcis or fasciola species
B peripheral blood eosinophilia, cholangitis and liver abscesses
C eventual progression to cholangiocarcinoma and biliary cirrhosis
D absence of abdominal pain or diarrhoea
E resistance to praziquantel therapy

117
Cestode infestation with *Taenia saginata* is associated with
A ingestion of undercooked pork
B abdominal pain and diarrhoea
C presentation with pruritus ani
D weight loss and malabsorption
E response to praziquantel therapy

118
Infestation with *Taenia solium* is typically associated with
A ingestion of undercooked fish
B liberation of larvae in the ileum from ingested ova
C larval penetration into the circulation via the stomach
D epilepsy and calcified cysts in skeletal muscle
E resistance to praziquantel therapy

119
Echinococcus granulosus infestation is usually associated with
A contact with sheep, cattle and dogs
B acquisition of hydatid cysts in childhood
C cysts in the liver, brain and lungs
D absence of dissemination during liver aspiration
E prompt response to albendazole therapy if surgically inoperable

---

Answers
113 A B D
114 A C D
115 A B D

116 A B
117 E
118 C D
119 A B C

120
In infestation with the nematode *Enterobius vermicularis*
A adult threadworms occur in great numbers in the small bowel
B presentation with intense pruritus ani is typical
C identifiable ova are found on the perianal skin
D malabsorption usually develops following heavy infestations
E all family members should take piperazine or mebendazole therapy

121
In infestation with *Ascaris lumbricoides*
A the disease follows ingestion of food contaminated with larvae
B larval migration through the lungs produces pulmonary eosinophilia
C obstruction of the ileum, biliary and pancreatic ducts occur
D malabsorption is the usual presentation
E levamisole in a single dose eradicates the disease

122
In infestation with *Trichuris trichura*
A weight loss and profuse watery diarrhoea are typical
B the ileum, caecum and colon are infested
C examination of the stool reveals visible whipworms
D pulmonary eosinophilia occurs during larval migration
E the therapy of choice is a single dose of oxantel

123
The typical features of ancylostomiasis include
A skin penetration with migration to the gut via the lungs
B hookworm parasitisation of the duodenum and jejunum
C pulmonary eosinophilia and haemoptysis
D iron deficiency anaemia and hypoproteinaemia
E eradication following mebendazole or pyrantel therapy

124
The typical features of strongyloidiasis include
A skin penetration with migration to the gut via the lungs
B larval penetration of the duodenal and jejunal mucosa
C abdominal pain, diarrhoea and malabsorption
D penetration of perianal skin producing a migrating linear weal
E systemic spread in the immunosuppressed resulting in pneumonia

125
The typical features of *Toxocara canis* infestation include
A larval penetration of the gastric mucosa
B asthma, pulmonary eosinophilia and splenomegaly
C development of the adult worms throughout the body tissues
D heavy infestation of the distal small bowel
E eradication with diethylcarbamazine therapy

Answers
120 B C E
121 B C E
122 B C E

123 A B C D E
124 A B C D E
125 A B E

126
The typical features of *Trichinella spiralis* infestation include
A infection resulting from contact with the urine of rodents
B larval migration from the small bowel to skeletal muscle
C oedema of the eyelids with muscle pain and tenderness
D acute myocarditis and encephalitis
E response to corticosteroid and thiabendazole therapy

127
In infection with *Wuchereria bancrofti*
A microfilaria are ingested in infected water
B lymphatic infiltration produces elephantiasis within a year
C epididymoorchitis, pleural effusions and ascites develop
D an incubation period of 2–4 weeks is typical
E treatment with diethylcarbamazine eradicates the disease

128
In infection with Loa loa
A transmission of microfilaria is by the mosquito *Culex fatigans*
B the incubation period is usually 3–12 days
C intermittent Calabar swellings in the subdermis are typical
D adult worms are visible traversing the eye beneath the conjunctiva
E diethylcarbamazine therapy is curative

129
In onchocerciasis
A larval infection is transmitted by the simulium fly
B worms mature over 2–4 weeks and persist for up to 1 year
C cutaneous nodules and eosinophilia commonly develop
D conjunctivitis, iritis and keratitis are characteristic
E diethylcarbamazine or ivermectin therapy are curative

130
Typical features of dracunculiasis include
A the ingestion of infected *Cyclops crustacea*
B larval penetration of the gut produces liver abscesses
C an incubation period of 9–18 weeks
D adult guinea worms rupture the skin to discharge their larvae
E therapy should include mebendazole and tetanus toxoid

Answers
126 B C D E
127 C E
128 C D E

129 A C D E
130 A D

Disturbances in water and electrolyte balance

1
In a normal 70 kg man, the following statements are true
A total body water is approximately 42 litres
B 70% of the total body water is intracellular
C 70% of extracellular water is intravascular
D sodium, bicarbonate and chloride ions are mainly intracellular
E potassium, magnesium, hydrogen, phosphate and sulphate ions are mainly extracellular

2
In a healthy man living in a temperate climate
A 500 ml of water per day are derived from metabolic processes
B water loss from the skin and lungs is about 250 ml per day
C obligatory urinary water loss is about 500 ml per day
D faecal water loss is about 500 ml per day
E urinary sodium losses can be reduced to less than 10 mmol per day in response to sodium depletion

3
Typical causes of sodium depletion include
A inadequate sodium intake
B prolonged use of diuretic drugs
C uncontrolled diabetes mellitus
D primary hypoadrenalism
E cystic fibrosis

4
Characteristic findings in predominant sodium depletion include
A thirst
B hypotension
C loss of skin turgor
D bradycardia
E muscle cramps

5
In the treatment of moderately severe sodium depletion
A the pulse and BP are reliable indices of severity and recovery
B 5% dextrose will help restore the extracellular fluid volume
C 2–4 L of isotonic saline should be given i.v. over 6–12 hours
D potassium and hydrogen ion balance are often disturbed
E isotonic sodium bicarbonate should be given in patients with a metabolic acidosis if there is pre-existing renal impairment

6
Primary water depletion is a recognised complication of
A primary hyperparathyroidism
B toxic confusional states
C oesophageal carcinoma
D lithium therapy
E acute pancreatitis

Answers
1 A B
2 A C E
3 B C D E

4 B C E
5 A C D E
6 A B C D

7
Expected features of severe primary water depletion include
A urine osmolality of 300 mosmol/kg
B plasma sodium of 130 mmol/L
C marked thirst and oliguria
D hypotension and peripheral circulatory failure
E muscle weakness and a "doughy" consistency of skin tissue

8
In the treatment of moderately severe water depletion
A the use of isotonic sodium chloride is contraindicated
B 5–10 L of isotonic dextrose should be given within 12–24 hours
C the urine volume reliably indicates the volume of fluid required
D cerebral oedema is the principal risk from hypotonic fluids
E the presence of peripheral circulatory failure suggests that a significant sodium depletion is also present

9
The following statements about potassium balance are true
A 85% of the daily potassium intake is excreted in the urine
B intracellular potassium ion concentrations are about 140 mmol/L
C cellular uptake of potassium is enhanced by adrenaline and insulin
D bicarbonate ions impair cellular uptake of potassium
E the normal potassium intake is about 2–3 g (50–80 mmol) per day

10
Recognised causes of potassium depletion include
A metabolic alkalosis
B cardiac failure
C hypertension
D renal tubular acidosis
E triamterene therapy

11
The clinical features of severe potassium depletion include
A polyuria due to renal tubular dysfunction
B muscle weakness, paraesthesiae and depressed tendon reflexes
C flattening of the T wave, ST depression and U waves on ECG
D abdominal distension and ileus
E sinus bradycardia and decreased digoxin sensitivity

12
Hyperkalaemia is a recognised finding in
A severe untreated diabetic ketoacidosis
B primary hypoadrenalism
C beta-blocker therapy in renal impairment
D prostaglandin inhibitor therapy in renal impairment
E angiotensin converting enzyme inhibitor therapy

13
Clinical features of hyperkalaemia include
A tall peaked T waves, ST depression and conduction defects on ECG
B asystole and ventricular fibrillation
C peripheral paraesthesiae
D prologation of the QT and widening of the QRS on ECG
E symptoms indistinguishable from those of hypokalaemia with muscle weakness, loss of tendon reflexes and ileus

14
The treatment of severe hyperkalaemia should include
A dietary restriction of coffee and fruit juices
B dextrose and glucagon i.v.
C calcium bicarbonate i.v.
D restoration of sodium and water balance
E calcium resonium orally and/or rectally

Answers
 7 C E
 8 A C D E
 9 A B C E
10 A B C D

11 A B C D
12 A B C D E
13 A B C D E
14 A D E

15
Magnesium deficiency
A causes confusion, depression and epilepsy
B is usually due to prolonged vomiting and diarrhoea
C is found in uncontrolled diabetes mellitus and alcoholism
D is found in primary hyperparathyroidism and hyperaldosteronism
E is best treated with magnesium sulphate given orally

16
The renal excretion of water is dependent on
A the glomerular filtration rate
B the proximal tubular reabsorption of solute
C solute concentrations in the ascending limb of the tubules
D the absence of anti-diuretic hormone (ADH)
E the integrity of the distal convoluted tubules

17
The following findings in acute water intoxication are to be expected
A serum sodium concentration < 130 mmol/L
B urinary osmolality 250 mosmol/kg
C nausea, headache and confusion
D prompt reponse to 1 litre of sodium chloride 0.9% i.v.
E increased ADH effect on renal collecting ducts with demeclocycline therapy

18
Inappropriate ADH secretion is reponsible for the dilutional hyponatraemia associated with the following
A addominal surgery
B meningoencephalitis
C hypothyroidism
D morphine and phenothiazine therapy
E chlorpropamide and carbamazepine therapy

19
Sodium and water retention should be expected following drug therapy with
A triamterene
B indomethacin
C oestrogens
D thyroxine
E captopril

20
The following statements about diuretic therapy are true
A frusemide reduces sodium reabsorption in the proximal tubules
B thiazides impair the renal excretion of glucose and uric acid
C triamterene antagonises aldosterone in the distal tubules
D amiloride is contraindicated in oliguric renal failure
E bumetanide can produce hyponatraemia even when oedema persists in severe cardiac, hepatic or renal failure

21
The following statements about hydrogen ion balance are true
A $[H^+] = k.[H_2CO_3]/[HCO_3^-]$
B the normal plasma hydrogen ion concentration is 36–44 nmol/L
C plasma bicarbonate is regulated solely by the renal tubules
D phosphoric and sulphuric acids are mainly excreted in the bile
E carbon dioxide is principally transported in the blood as carbaminohaemoglobin

Answers
15 A B C D
16 A B C D E
17 A C
18 A B D

19 B C
20 D E
21 A B C

22
The following statements about the assessment of acid-base balance in healthy subjects are true

A the blood pH is derived from the measured arterial $PaCO_2$

B the urinary ammonium concentration is a measure of blood pH

C the anion gap, expressed as $[Na^+] + [K^+] - [Cl^-] - [HCO_3^-]$), is < 15 mmol/L

D the blood $PaCO_2$ correlates closely with alveolar $PaCO_2$

E the 'standard bicarbonate' is the bicarbonate concentration corrected for a standard $PaCO_2$ of 4.3 kPa

23
Characteristic findings in the metabolic acidosis associated with the following conditions include

A increased plasma bicarbonate concentration in lactic acidosis

B decreased urinary hydrogen ion concentration in renal failure

C increased blood $PaCO_2$ in diabetic ketoacidosis

D low plasma chloride concentration in renal tubular acidosis

E increased red cell carbonic acid production during acetazolamide therapy

24
Given a PaO_2 6 kPa, $PaCO_2$ 5.5, $[H^+]$ 60 nmol/L and actual $[HCO_3^-]$ 23 mmol/L, the following statements are true

A salicylate poisoning should be considered likely

B cardiac arrest alone would produce similar blood gases

C severe diarrhoea alone would produce similar blood gases

D diabetic ketoacidosis alone would produce similar blood gases

E the picture suggests that the blood gas results are erroneous

25
The following statements about the treatment of metabolic acidosis in diabetic ketoacidosis are true

A 1.26% sodium bicarbonate should be given if acidosis is severe

B 0.9% sodium chloride is indicated to correct sodium depletion

C in renal impairment, sodium bicarbonate is contraindicated

D the serum potassium is an unreliable marker of total body potassium

E total sodium losses are usually less than 200 mmol

26
Characteristic findings in metabolic alkalosis due to prolonged vomiting include

A arterial $PaCO_2$ 6 kPa, $[H^+]$ 25 nmol/L, actual $[HCO_3^-]$ 34 mmol/L

B urinary pH 5 with proteinuria and renal tubular casts

C increased renal tubular sodium and potassium reabsorption

D increased plasma chloride and potassium concentrations

E increased plasma ionised calcium concentration

27
The following statements about respiratory acidosis (RAC) and respiratory alkalosis (RAK) are true

A renal tubular bicarbonate reabsorption is enhanced in RAC

B salicylate poisoning produces both RAK and metabolic acidosis

C an arterial $PaCO_2$ 3 kPa and $[H^+]$ 30 nmol/L suggests RAK

D pulmonary embolism should be suspected if RAC is present

E electrolyte solutions should be started promptly in the treatment of both RAC and RAK

Answers
22 B C D
23 B
24 none

25 A B D
26 A B
27 A B C

Oncology

1
The following factors are associated aetiologically with the carcinomas listed below
A malignant melanoma — coffee consumption
B cervical carcinoma — chlamydial infection
C hepatocellular carcinoma — hepatitis B infection
D pancreatic carcinoma — alcohol consumption
E oesophageal carcinoma — tobacco consumption

2
Tumour markers associated with the following diseases include
A human chorionic gonadotrophin — testicular seminoma
B alpha-foetoprotein — primary hepatocellular carcinoma
C carcinoembryonic antigen — bronchial adenoma
D placental alkaline phosphatase — cervical carcinoma
E prolactin inhibitory factor — breast carcinoma

3
The following statements about the predictive value (PV) of a screening test are true
A PV is dependent on the prevalence of the disease under review
B PV is dependent on the test's sensitivity but not its specificity
C sensitivity is inversely related to specificity
D specificity = %(+ ve) tests of all patients with the disease
E sensitivity = %(- ve) tests of all subjects free of the disease

4
The paraneoplastic syndromes listed below are recognised associations of the following tumours
A ADH activity — adenocarcinoma of lung
B parathyroid hormone activity — squamous cell carcinoma of lung
C polymyositis — breast carcinoma
D myasthenia-like syndrome — small cell lung carcinoma
E acanthosis nigricans — gastric carcinoma

Answers
1 C D E
2 B

3 C
4 B C D E

41

5
The following statements about the clinical staging of tumours and evaluation of the response to therapy are correct
A the TNM system defines tumour size and the number of metastases
B T0 indicates undetectable tumour proven only by aspirate cytology
C Dukes' B classification of pancreatic carcinoma = < 5 cm in size
D a partial response to therapy = > 50% reduction in tumour size
E Stage IIb Ann Arbor classification of Non-Hodgkin gastric lymphoma indicates disease on both sides of the diaphragm

6
In the Ann Arbor staging of lymphomas
A intra-thoracic and intra-abdominal lymphadenopathy = stage III
B splenomegaly and intra-abdominal lymphadenopathy = stage IIIS
C diffuse hepatic or bone marrow involvement = stage IV
D gastric and splenic involvement = IISE
E pulmonary hilar lymphadenopathy with fever = stage IB

7
In the TNM staging of bronchial carcinoma
A TX indicates positive cytology
B T2 indicates tumour size > 3 cm and/or extension to hilar nodes
C malignant pleural effusion would be staged as T4
D N1 indicates extension to the ipsilateral mediastinum
E M0 indicates the absence of metastases

8
The following statements about radiotherapy are true
A ionising radiation damages cell nuclear DNA
B 1 Gray of absorbed radiation = 1 Joule per kilogram of tissue
C brachytherapy is radiotherapy delivered by an external beam
D megavoltage teletherapy is used for skin tumours
E hypoxia enhances tissue sensitivity to irradiation

9
The following statements about chemotherapy are true
A methotrexate is an anti-folate blocking nucleotide synthesis
B azathioprine is an alkylating agent blocking DNA transcription
C adriamycin is a plant alkaloid which disrupts mitotic spindles
D cisplatin is a nitrosourea which blocks pyrimidine synthesis
E melphalan is an alkylating agent which blocks DNA replication

10
The general principles governing the use of combination chemotherapy include
A the toxic effects of each drug should be closely similar
B each drug should have a similar mode of action
C each drug should be of proven efficacy individually
D drugs used in combination should not have adverse interactions
E the minimum effective dose of each drug should be used

Answers
5 D
6 ACD E
7 ABCE

8 A B
9 A E
10 C D

11
Malignant diseases known to be potentially curable following appropriate combination chemotherapy include
A malignant melanoma
B myelomatosis
C choriocarcinoma
D anaplastic thyroid carcinoma
E Hodgkin's lymphoma

12
Malignant diseases known to be refractory to current chemotherapeutic agents include
A squamous cell bronchial carcinoma
B oesophageal carcinoma
C colorectal carcinoma
D ovarian carcinoma
E malignant melanoma

13
The following adverse effects are associated with the use of the chemotherapy drugs listed below
A alopecia — cyclophosphamide
B acute leukaemia — methotrexate
C cardiomyopathy — adriamycin
D pulmonary fibrosis — cisplatin
E neuropathy — vincristine

14
The following endocrine therapies are of proven value in the therapy of the malignant diseases listed below
A gonadotrophin releasing hormone — prostatic carcinoma
B thyroxine — papillary thyroid carcinoma
C progesterone — endometrial carcinoma
D aminoglutethamide — testicular teratoma
E tamoxifen — breast carcinoma

Answers
11 C E
12 A B C E

13 A C E
14 A B C E

Diseases of the cardiovascular system

1

The pain of myocardial ischaemia

A is typically induced by exercise and relieved by rest

B radiates to the neck and jaw but not the teeth

C rarely lasts longer than 10 seconds after resting

D is easily distinguished from oesophageal pain

E can disappear if exercise is continued

2

Syncope

A followed by facial flushing suggests a tachyarrhythmia

B without warning suggests a vaso-vagal episode

C on exercise is a typical feature of mitral incompetence

D on coughing is due to a reflex bradyarrhythmia

E due to glyceryl trinitrate is improved by beta-blockade

3

Typical features of severe cardiac failure include

A tiredness

B nocturia

C anorexia and epigastric pain

D hyperpnoea

E nocturnal cough

4

In a patient with nocturnal dyspnoea, the clinical features useful in distinguishing left ventricular failure from an exacerbation of chronic bronchitis include

A orthopnoea

B peripheral cyanosis

C basal crepitations

D sinus tachycardia

E blood-stained sputum

5

In a patient with suspected heart disease

A stabbing inframammary pain is likely to be cardiac in origin

B effort dyspnoea is unequivocal evidence of cardiac failure

C palpitation disappearing on exertion suggests an ischaemic origin

D the absence of symptoms excludes serious disease

E central cyanosis is indicative of a reduced cardiac output

6

The following pulse characteristics are typical features of the disorders listed below

A pulsus bisferiens — combined mitral stenosis and incompetence

B pulsus paradoxus — aortic incompetence

C collapsing pulse — severe anaemia

D pulsus alternans — extrasystoles every alternate beat

E anacrotic pulse — hypertrophic cardiomyopathy

Answers

1 A E

2 none

3 A B C E

4 B E

5 none

6 C

7
During the Valsalva manoeuvre
A an increase in the pulse rate suggests left ventricular failure
B forced inspiration is undertaken against a closed glottis
C the blood pressure falls due to a reflex bradycardia
D mitral murmurs are initially accentuated
E the blood pressure and pulse rate normally rise soon after straining is terminated

8
The following statements about the jugular venous pulse (JVP) are true
A the JVP should be measured with the patient reclining at 25°
B a JVP < 3 cm above the suprasternal notch is normal
C the JVP, unlike the blood pressure, does not rise with anxiety
D the JVP does not normally rise on abdominal compression
E the JVP in normal subjects falls during inspiration

9
Components of the jugular venous pulse are explained on the basis of the following physiological events
A 'c' wave = closure of the tricuspid valve
B 'a' wave = atrial systole
C 'v' wave = onset of ventricular systole
D 'x' descent = atrial relaxation
E 'y' descent = ventricular diastole and tricuspid valve opening

10
The following abnormalities of the jugular venous pulse are associated with the disorders listed below
A cannon waves = pulmonary hypertension
B giant 'a' waves = AV dissociation
C 'cv' waves = tricuspid incompetence
D prominent 'y' descent = constrictive pericarditis
E prominent 'x' descent = tricuspid stenosis

11
Characteristic abnormalities on palpation of the cardiac impulse are associated with the following disorders
A 'tapping' apex = right ventricular hypertrophy
B left parasternal heave = right ventricular hypertrophy
C left parasternal systolic thrill = mitral incompetence
D impalpable apex beat = emphysema
E upper sternal lift = thoracic aortic aneurysm

12
The following heart sounds (S_1, S_2, S_3, S_4) are associated with the phenomena shown below
A third heart sound = rapid ventricular filling
B loud first heart sound = long P-R interval on ECG
C soft first heart sound = mitral stenosis
D single second heart sound = Fallot's tetralogy
E fourth heart sound = atrial fibrillation

13
Abnormalities of the second heart sound (S_2) are associated with the following cardiac disorders
A fixed splitting = complete right bundle branch block
B reversed splitting = complete left bundle branch block
C absence of splitting = hypertrophic cardiomyopathy
D palpable second heart sound = pulmonary hypertension
E splitting only during inspiration = physiological splitting

14
A third heart sound (S_3) is a typical finding in
A mitral stenosis
B healthy young athletes
C constrictive pericarditis
D tricuspid incompetence
E left ventricular dyskinesia

Answers
   7 none
   8 E
   9 B D E
  10 C D

  11 B D E
  12 A D
  13 B D E
  14 B C D E

15
The following statements about cardiac murmurs are true
A diastolic murmurs are a recognised feature of normal pregnancy
B ventricular septal defects produce pansystolic murmurs
C an early high-pitched diastolic murmur suggests mitral stenosis
D late-systolic murmurs suggest mitral valve prolapse
E mitral diastolic murmurs are best heard at the apex with the patient leaning forwards and the breath held in expiration

16
The following statements indicate that a regular tachycardia is ventricular rather than supraventricular in origin
A a ventricular rate > 160/minute
B irregular cannon waves
C variable intensity of the first heart sound (S_1)
D the presence of cardiac failure
E QRS complexes < 0.14 sec in duration on ECG

17
The following statements about sphygmomanometry in the measurement of the blood pressure (BP) are true
A an arm cuff smaller than recommended lowers the BP recording
B appearance of the first Korotkov sound denotes systolic pressure
C muffling of the sound denotes phase V diastolic pressure
D inter-observer variation is less with phase IV than phase V
E the resting BP correlates more closely with cardiovascular risk than random BP recordings

18
In the normal resting cardiac cell, the electrical potential difference across the cell membrane
A is principally attributable to the potassium gradient
B depolarises in response to the rapid influx of sodium
C depolarises in response to the slow influx of calcium
D repolarises by cessation of the calcium influx
E is maintained by a sodium pump which preserves a higher intracellular than extracellular sodium concentration

19
The following statements about the nature and polarity of the classical leads used in a 12-lead ECG are true
A the earth lead is attached to the right leg
B lead 1 = left arm positive with respect to the right arm
C lead 11 = left leg positive with respect to the right arm
D aVR = right arm positive with respect to both legs
E V_2 = second intercostal space at the left sternal edge with respect to the electrode connecting both arms and one leg

20
In the normal ECG, depolarisation
A of the atria is recorded as the P wave
B of the interventricular septum is recorded by the Q wave in V_5-V_6
C proceeds from epicardium to endocardium
D of the endocardium produces the T wave
E voltage amplitudes vary with the thickness of cardiac muscle

---

Answers
15 B D
16 B C
17 B

18 A B D
19 A B C
20 A B E

21
In the investigation of patients with cardiac failure
A the cardiothoracic ratio (CTR) on chest X ray is usually > 0.6
B pulmonary venous congestion is the earliest change on chest X ray
C two-dimensional echocardiography can estimate cardiac output
D Doppler echocardiography can estimate pressure gradients
E radionuclide myocardial scanning can identify areas of ischaemia

22
The following statements about cardiac rhythms are true
A cardiac rate falls with inspiration in autonomic neuropathy
B re-entry tachyarrhythmias arise from anomalous AV conduction
C sinus bradycardia < 60/min is a normal occurrence during sleep
D sinus arrest is defined on ECG by P waves without QRS complexes
E sick sinus syndrome is characterised by episodes of both bradycardias and tachycardias associated with sinus node disease

23
The following features are characteristically associated with supraventricular tachycardias (SVT)
A underlying cardiac disease when cardiac failure is present
B cardiac rate of 160–220/minute in young, asymptomatic patients
C polyuria following prolonged episodes
D proptosis when thyrotoxicosis is present
E bundle branch block on ECG when the cardiac rate > 180/min

24
Typical features of the Wolff-Parkinson-White (WPW) syndrome include
A tachyarrythmias as a result of a re-entry phenomenon
B ventricular pre-excitation via an accessory AV pathway
C atrial fibrillation with a ventricular response of > 160/min
D long P-R interval and narrow QRS complex on ECGs between bouts
E therapeutic response to beta-blockade and/or digoxin

25
Atrial tachycardia with AV block is characteristically associated with
A an irregularly irregular pulse
B slowing of the atrial rate on carotid sinus massage
C the absence of underlying cardiac disease
D digoxin toxicity and intracellular potassium depletion
E a poor response to digoxin therapy in patients who have not previously been taking digoxin

26
In atrial flutter
A the radial pulse is usually regular or regularly irregular
B carotid sinus massage slows the AV conduction
C the heart is usually otherwise normal
D the atrial rate is about 240/minute
E digoxin often converts the rhythm to atrial fibrillation

27
In atrial fibrillation
A patients are invariably symptomatic
B the radial pulse is totally irregular
C the cardiac output falls due to the absence of atrial systole
D cardioversion is contraindicated during anticoagulant therapy
E alcohol abuse is a recognised cause

Answers
21 B D E
22 B C E
23 A C E

24 A B C
25 D
26 A B E
27 B C E

28
Ventricular ectopic beats
A can be distinguished from atrial extrasystoles on auscultation
B usually occur at fixed intervals following the sinus beat
C in cardiac disease usually disappear on exercise
D occur as escape beats given an underlying bradycardia
E following acute myocardial infarction should be treated with lignocaine to prevent ventricular fibrillation

29
In ventricular tachycardia (VT)
A underlying cardiac disease is usually present
B symptoms are invariably more severe than those of an SVT
C a shortened QT interval on ECG predisposes to recurrent VT
D carotid sinus massage usually slows the rate transiently
E associated with cardiac failure, cardioversion should be avoided

30
In ventricular fibrillation
A the radial pulse is usually extremely rapid and thready
B the patient is always unconscious prior to resuscitation
C ECG confirmation is vital before DC shock is administered
D cardioversion should be synchronised with the R wave on ECG
E lignocaine therapy given at the onset should abort the arrhythmia

31
When instituting cardiopulmonary resuscitation (CPR) following the onset of cardiac arrest
A a sharp blow to the praecordium can restore sinus rhythm
B the commonest underlying arrhythmia is asystole
C iv sodium bicarbonate should be given to avert metabolic acidosis
D intracardiac adrenaline should be given if cardioversion fails
E with only one operator CPR is best achieved by inflating the lungs twice then delivering 15 sternal compressions at 80/min

32
The therapeutic actions of digoxin include
A shortening the refractory period of conducting tissue
B lengthening the refractory period of cardiac muscle
C potentiation of effect by hyperkalaemia
D inhibitory drug interaction with concomitant quinidine therapy
E risk of ventricular fibrillation in patients on digoxin undergoing cardioversion

33
Digoxin
A is indicated in most patients with atrial fibrillation
B usually converts atrial flutter to sinus rhythm
C acts primarily on cell membrane ionic pumps
D self-poisoning can be treated with drug-specific antibodies
E -induced ventricular tachyarrhythmias are best treated with verapamil

---

Answers
28 B D
29 A
30 B

31 A E
32 E
33 A C D

34
Drugs indicated in the long-term prophylaxis of supraventricular tachycardias include
A mexiletine
B nifedipine
C digoxin
D amiodarone
E procainamide

35
Drugs indicated in the long-term prophylaxis of ventricular tachycardias include
A verapamil
B amiodarone
C lignocaine
D mexiletine
E sotalol

36
In the classification of anti-arrhythmic drugs, the following statements are true
A Class I agents increase the effective refractory period
B Class II agents inhibit the slow calcium channel
C Class III agents inhibit the fast sodium channel
D Class IV agents antagonise beta-adrenoceptors
E phenytoin accelerates conduction in Purkinje fibres by increasing the initial rapid phase (0) of the action potential

37
Class I anti-arrhythmic drugs exhibit the following features
A Class Ia drugs like disopyramide increase the QT interval
B Class Ia drugs slow conduction in atrial and ventricular muscle
C Class Ia drugs have anti-cholinergic effects
D Class Ib drugs like lignocaine are excreted by the kidneys
E Class Ib drugs should only be given intravenously

38
The following Class II anti-arrhythmic drugs selectively block the beta$_1$ adrenoreceptor
A sotalol
B atenolol
C acebutolol
D metoprolol
E timolol

39
The following statements about Class III anti-arrhythmic drugs are true
A they prolong the plateau phase of the action potential
B both sotalol and disopyramide have Class II activity
C amiodarone is useful in the prevention of VT but not SVT
D amiodarone should be withdrawn if corneal deposits occur
E amiodarone has a plasma half-life of 30 days and interacts significantly with both digoxin and warfarin therapy

40
The following statements about Class IV anti-arrhythmic drugs are true
A nifedipine slows AV conduction and lowers the blood pressure
B verapamil is useful in distinguishing SVT from VT
C all Class IV drugs should be avoided in cardiac failure
D verapamil should be avoided in atrial fibrillation
E all Class IV drugs reduce both preload and afterload

Answers
34 C D
35 B D E
36 A E
37 A B C

38 B C D
39 A B E
40 C

41
The following statements about atrioventricular (AV) block are true
A first degree block is associated with a loud first heart sound
B the PR interval can be fixed or variable in second degree block
C decreasing PR intervals suggests Wenckebach's phenomenon
D irregular cannon waves in the JVP suggests complete heart block
E the radial pulse is typically slow but regularly irregular when third degree (complete) heart block occurs in atrial fibrillation

42
Absolute indications for permanent endocardial pacing include
A asymptomatic congenital complete heart block
B asymptomatic second degree heart block
C Stokes-Adams attacks in the elderly
D complete heart block in rheumatic mitral valve disease
E symptomatic second degree heart block following acute inferior myocardial infarction

43
The following statements about complete bundle branch block (BBB) are true
A CRBBB can result from left ventricular hypertrophy
B CRBBB produces right axis deviation with a QRS > 0.12 sec on ECG
C CRBBB produces reversed splitting of the second heart sound
D CLBBB produces fixed splitting of the second heart sound
E damage to the posterior limb of the left bundle (left posterior hemiblock) produces left axis deviation on ECG

44
Typical clinical features of acute circulatory failure include
A periodic respiration
B renal vasoconstriction
C central cyanosis
D confusion
E thirst and polyuria

45
Acute circulatory failure with an elevated central venous pressure would be an expected finding in
A acute pancreatitis
B massive pulmonary embolism
C ruptured ectopic pregnancy
D acute right ventricular infarction
E pericardial tamponade

46
The following would be typical findings in a previously fit 40 year old man after losing 1 litre of blood over two hours
A radial pulse 130/min and systolic blood pressure < 100 mmHg
B mean left atrial pressure > 10 mmHg
C urine output of 50 ml per hour
D urinary sodium concentration of 20 mmol/L
E haemoglobin concentration of 10 g/dL

47
In the treatment of cardiac failure associated with acute pulmonary oedema
A 28% oxygen should be administered using a Ventimask
B morphine reduces angor animi, preload and afterload
C iv frusemide produces an immediate reduction in preload
D nitrates reduce the afterload to improve ventricular efficiency
E ACE inhibitors decrease the afterload but increase the preload

Answers
41 B D
42 C D
43 none
44 A B D
45 B D E
46 none
47 B C

52 Diseases of the cardiovascular system

48
The following therapies produce their main cardiovascular effects in the manner described below
A alpha$_1$ blockers act to reduce the afterload
B calcium antagonists act to reduce the preload
C dopamine acts on dopamine receptor mediating vasoconstriction
D dobutamine acts on beta$_1$ receptor with chronotropic effects
E positive-pressure ventilation can be useful in acute pulmonary oedema of cardiac origin by reducing right ventricular output

49
Right ventricular hypertrophy is an expected finding in adults with the following longstanding disorders
A tricuspid stenosis
B constrictive pericarditis
C cor pulmonale
D atrial septal defect
E mitral stenosis

50
Left ventricular hypertrophy is an expected finding in adults with the following longstanding disorders
A mitral stenosis
B aortic stenosis
C Addison's disease
D left atrial myxoma
E hypertrophic cardiomyopathy

51
In chronic biventricular cardiac failure
A glomerular filtration rate falls lowering the plasma renin
B excess ADH causes oedema to develop
C hyponatraemia and hypokalaemia indicate total body depletion
D prothrombin synthesis is usually normal
E diuretic requirements are usually less in mobile patients than patients on bed rest

52
The following features would be expected in cardiac failure
A development at the onset of atrial fibrillation in mitral stenosis
B weight loss due to anorexia
C predominantly lower lobe pulmonary venous congestion
D satisfactory response to nitrate therapy in aortic stenosis
E adverse response to nitrate therapy in mitral stenosis

53
In addition to evidence of a recent streptococcal infection, the diagnosis of acute rheumatic fever is confirmed by
A fever with an elevated erythrocyte sedimentation rate
B arthralgia and a previous history of rheumatic fever
C chorea and a prolonged PR interval on ECG
D erythema nodosum and arthritis
E rheumatic nodules and pancarditis

54
The following are typical features of acute rheumatic fever
A recent infection with Group B haemolytic streptococci
B transient pink patches on the trunk enlarging to form crescents
C tachycardia with a loud first heart sound
D transient mid-diastolic murmur
E symmetrical polyarthritis of the PIP and MCP joints

Answers
48 E
49 C D E
50 B E
51 none

52 A B E
53 E
54 B D

55
In the management and prognosis of acute rheumatic fever
A aspirin improves the long-term prognosis
B antibiotics should be given until the age 13 years
C prednisolone improves the long-term prognosis
D chronic valvular heart disease is likely if chorea is present
E if pericarditis is present, myocarditis can also be assumed to be present and the risk of chronic valvular disease is > 90%

56
In patients with severe mitral stenosis
A the mitral valve orifice is reduced from 5 cm^2 to about 1 cm^2
B a history of rheumatic fever or chorea is elicited in over 90%
C pulmonary hypertension is more marked if sinus rhythm is present
D the risk of systemic emboli is trivial if sinus rhythm is present
E mitral valvotomy is indicated if the valve is pliant and incompetent

57
Features suggesting a calcified mitral valve associated with atrial fibrillation, mitral stenosis and incompetence include
A soft apical mid-systolic and early diastolic murmurs
B cough, breathlessness and haemoptysis
C left parasternal heave and a heaving, displaced apex beat
D giant A waves in the JVP and both third and fourth heart sounds
E soft first heart sound, absent opening snap and loud second heart sound

58
The clinical features of mitral valve prolapse include
A mid-systolic click and late-systolic murmur
B auscultatory findings which vary with posture
C an association in young adults with embolic stroke
D predisposition to tachyarrhythmias
E predisposition to infective endocarditis

59
Recognised features of chronic mitral incompetence include
A soft first heart sound and short mid-diastolic murmur
B onset associated with congestive cardiomyopathy
C afterload reduction increases the severity of regurgitation
D pansystolic murmur and heaving, displaced apex beat
E atrial fibrillation requiring anticoagulation

60
Disorders typically producing the sudden onset of symptomatic mitral incompetence include
A Marfan's syndrome
B acute myocardial infarction
C acute rheumatic fever
D infective endocarditis
E diphtheria

61
Clinical features suggesting severe aortic stenosis include
A late-systolic ejection click
B pulsus bisferiens
C heaving, displaced apex beat
D syncope associated with angina
E loud second heart sound

Answers
55 D
56 A C
57 B C E

58 A B C D E
59 A B D
60 B C D E
61 C D

62
Disorders associated with aortic incompetence include
A ankylosing spondylitis
B Marfan's syndrome
C syphilitic aortitis
D persistent ductus arteriosus
E Takayasu disease

63
Typical clinical features of aortic incompetence include
A anterior mitral valve flutter on echocardiography
B diastolic thrill at the left sternal edge
C left parasternal heave and displaced apex beat
D collapsing pulse with pulsatile nailbed capillaries
E mid-systolic murmur usually indicating aortic stenosis rather than merely the result of an increased stroke volume

64
The following statements about tricuspid valve disease are true
A murmurs are best heard in mid-sternum at the end of expiration
B ascites can occur from incompetence but not stenosis
C in sinus rhythm, stenosis produces cannon waves in the JVP
D both stenosis and incompetence produce a pulsatile liver
E tricuspid stenosis or incompetence due to rheumatic heart disease is invariably associated with mitral valve disease

65
The typical features of congenital pulmonary stenosis include
A breathlessness and central cyanosis
B giant A waves in the JVP
C loud second heart sound preceded by an ejection systolic click
D left parasternal heave and systolic thrill
E gradient of 60 mmHg across the outflow tract indicates severe disease requiring intervention

66
In infective endocarditis
A streptococci and staphylococci account for over 80% of cases
B stenotic rather than incompetent valves are more often involved
C normal cardiac valves are not affected
D glomerulonephritis usually occurs due to immune complex disease
E the cardinal features are fever, emboli and changing murmurs

67
In the management of infective endocarditis
A three sets of blood cultures are sufficient to establish the cause
B antibiotic therapy should await bacteriological confirmation
C parenteral antibiotic therapy should be continued for 6 weeks
D probenecid should routinely accompany penicillin therapy
E cardiac surgery should be considered if the valve affected is prosthetic or if there is progressive cardiac failure

68
The normal right coronary artery
A supplies the inferior aspect of the left ventricle
B supplies the AV node
C divides into the circumflex and marginal arteries
D supplies the right ventricle and part of the septum
E arises from the left sinus of Valsalva

Answers
62 A B C
63 A D
64 E
65 B D

66 A D E
67 A D E
68 A B D

69
The normal left coronary artery
A supplies the anterior and apical parts of the left ventricle
B divides into the anterior descending and circumflex arteries
C supplies part of the interventricular septum
D arises from the left sinus of Valsalva
E supplies the lateral and posterior parts of the left ventricle from the circumflex artery

70
In the investigation of suspected angina pectoris
A the resting ECG is usually abnormal
B exercise-induced elevation in BP indicates significant ischaemia
C a normal ECG during exercise excludes angina pectoris
D coronary angiography is indicated if an exercise test is normal
E coronary artery surgery improves survival in asymptomatic patients with triple vessel disease

71
In the treatment of patients with angina pectoris
A lowering a high plasma cholesterol has no effect on survival
B regular exercise should be avoided if angina occurs daily
C nitrate-induced tachycardia usually persists despite beta blockade
D nifedipine is a potent systemic and coronary arteriolar dilator
E cardio-selective beta blockers are more effective than non-selective beta blockers especially in variant angina

72
Angina pectoris is a recognised feature of
A anaemia without underlying coronary artery disease
B polyarteritis nodosa
C ventricular but not supraventricular tachyarrhythmias
D aortic stenosis
E Monckeberg's medial sclerosis

73
In a patient with central chest pain, the diagnosis of angina pectoris is likely given the following features
A burning retrosternal pain in the early evening
B waking from sleep with nocturnal pain and angor animi
C exercise-induced pain relieved within 5 minutes by rest
D left-sided anterior chest wall tenderness
E exercise ECG changes with > 2mm ST depression without chest pain

74
The diagnosis of acute myocardial infarction is supported by the following features
A nausea and vomiting
B breathlessness and angor animi
C hypotension and peripheral cyanosis
D tiredness and pallor
E pleuritic central chest pain

75
Typical findings consistent with an acute anterior myocardial infarction occurring within the previous six hours include
A hypertension and raised JVP
B pericardial friction rub
C ST elevation > 2mm in leads II, III and aVF on ECG
D gallop rhythm and soft first heart sound
E serum LDH > 3000 iu/L

Answers
69 A B C D E
70 none
71 D

72 B D
73 B C E
74 A B C D E
75 A D

76
Following an acute myocardial infarction
A an initial fall in BP is commoner than a rise in BP
B an exercise ECG should be deferred for at least 3 months
C survivors of VF have reduced survival rates
D cardiac failure and heart block both augur a poor prognosis
E pleuritic chest pain and fever occurring within 3 days usually indicates pulmonary infarction

77
Recognised consequences of acute myocardial infarction include
A persistently elevated JVP without left ventricular failure
B atrial fibrillation association with a bradycardia
C ventricular septal defect
D revoking of the patient's HGV driving licence
E persistent fever, pericarditis and pleural effusions

78
In the treatment of acute myocardial infarction
A aspirin given within six hours of onset reduces the mortality
B i.v. streptokinase reduces infarct size and mortality by > 25%
C diamorphine is best given iv than by any other route
D immediate beta blockade reduces the initial mortality rate
E digoxin should be avoided for supraventricular tachyarrhythmias

79
In the treatment of arrhythmias following acute myocardial infarction
A atropine should be given for all sinus bradycardias
B frequent ventricular ectopics usually require i.v. lignocaine
C complete heart block in inferior infarcts requires a pacemaker
D i.v. lignocaine should immediately precede cardioversion for VF
E cardioversion should be considered as first-line therapy for most tachyarrhythmias if cardiac failure or hypotension supervene

80
The following statements about the prognosis of acute myocardial infarction are true
A 40% of all patients die within 1 month of whom 75% die on day 1
B beta blockade improves a patient's survival at 1 year by 25%
C stress and social isolation adversely affect the prognosis
D reducing a high plasma cholesterol improves the survival at 1 year
E on average, survivors have a 75% chance of living for 5 years, 50% for 10 years and 25% for 20 years

81
The following statements about systemic hypertension are true
A casual BP recordings correlate poorly with life expectancy
B systolic hypertension alone is of little prognostic value
C most patients have a normal plasma renin concentration
D 15% of the adult UK population have essential hypertension
E 15% of hypertensives have hypertension secondary to other disorders of whom 70% have a family history of hypertension

---

Answers
76 D
77 A B C D E
78 A B C

79 E
80 A C E
81 C D

82
Recognised causes of secondary hypertension include
A persistent ductus arteriosus
B primary hyperaldosteronism
C acromegaly
D pregnancy and oestrogen therapy
E thyrotoxicosis

83
In patients with systemic hypertension, the following provide important aetiological clues
A symmetrical small joint polyarthritis
B radio-femoral delay in the pulses
C smell of alcohol on the breath
D epigastric bruit
E palpably enlarged kidneys

84
Complications of systemic hypertension include
A retinal microaneurysms
B dissecting aneurysm of the ascending aorta
C renal artery stenosis
D lacunar strokes of the internal capsule
E subdural haemorrhage

85
In the investigation of systemic hypertension
A hyperkalaemic metabolic acidosis indicates hyperaldosteronism
B excretion urography is necessary to exclude renal artery stenosis
C normal urinary 5-HIAA excretion should exclude phaeochromocytoma
D urine analysis for blood, protein and glucose is essential
E radionuclide renography is best undertaken before treatment with an ACE inhibitor

86
Accelerated phase or malignant hypertension is indicated by
A loud second heart sound
B heaving apex beat
C diastolic BP > 130 mmHg
D retinal soft exudates or papilloedema
E renal or cardiac failure

87
In the emergency treatment of malignant hypertension
A therapy should reduce the BP < *150/90* mmHg within 30 minutes
B when indicated, iv nitroprusside is best administered rapidly
C ACE inhibitors are ideal given bilateral renal artery stenosis
D vasodilator therapy to reduce the afterload should be used
E in renal failure, a beta blocker is often the drug of choice

88
In the treatment of mild – moderate systemic hypertension
A treatment reduces mortality in patients with mild hypertension
B alcohol, stress and calorie reduction can all lower the BP
C moderating salt intake is as important as avoidance of smoking
D thiazides are better tolerated in the elderly than beta blockade
E an initial hypotensive reaction following the introduction of an ACE inhibitor is particularly common in sodium-depleted patients

89
Hypertension refractory to medical therapy requires exclusion of the following possibilities
A inadequate drug therapy
B poor drug compliance
C phaeochromocytoma
D anti-inflammatory drug therapy
E renal artery stenosis

Answers
82 B C D
83 A B C D E
84 C D
85 D

86 C D E
87 D
88 B D E
89 A B C D E

90
Recognised causes of pulmonary arterial hypertension include
A mitral stenosis
B atrial septal defect
C chronic bronchitis
D pulmonary thromboembolism
E persistent ductus arteriosus

91
Typical clinical features of primary pulmonary hypertension include
A male preponderance
B exertional syncope
C systemic arterial emboli
D giant A waves in the JVP and right parasternal heave
E loud second heart sound and early diastolic murmur

92
Clinical features characteristic of massive pulmonary embolism include
A central and peripheral cyanosis
B pleuritic chest pain and haemoptysis
C breathlessness and syncope
D tachycardia and elevated JVP
E abnormal chest X-ray and Q waves in leads I, II and aVL on ECG

93
Recognised features of pulmonary infarction include
A peripheral blood leucocytosis and fever
B pleuro-pericardial friction rub
C blood-stained pleural effusion
D development of a lung abscess
E ipsilateral elevation of the hemidiaphragm

94
In the treatment of acute pulmonary thromboembolism
A streptokinase therapy reduces mortality more than heparin alone
B 28% oxygen therapy should maintain the $PaO_2 > 12$ kPa
C diamorphine should be avoided if the patient is severely hypoxic
D the heparin infusion should continue until day 1 of warfarin therapy
E warfarin therapy should be continued for three weeks

95
Recognised causes of dilated (congestive) cardiomyopathy include
A systemic lupus erythematosus
B haemochromatosis
C sarcoidosis
D chronic alcohol abuse
E thyrotoxicosis

96
Recognised causes of restrictive (obliterative) cardiomyopathy include
A acromegaly
B Addison's disease
C amyloidosis
D hypereosinophilic syndrome
E tropical endocardial fibrosis

97
Clinical features compatible with a cardiomyopathy include
A absence of a previous history of angina or myocardial infarction
B absence of cardiac arrhythmias
C biventricular dilatation with an ejection fraction < 20%
D dyskinetic segment of left ventricle on echocardiography
E functional mitral incompetence

Answers
90 A B C D E
91 B D E
92 A C D
93 A B C D E

94 none
95 A B C D E
96 C D E
97 A C E

98
Clinical features compatible with hypertrophic cardiomyopathy include
A family history of Friedreich's ataxia or sudden death
B angina pectoris and exertional syncope
C jerky pulse and heaving apex beat
D murmurs suggesting both aortic stenosis and mitral incompetence
E syncope improved by beta blockade but exacerbated by digoxin or calcium antagonists

99
In acute pericarditis
A chest pain is typically like the pain of myocardial infarction
B the friction rub is best heard at the apex in mid-expiration
C friction rubs invariably disappear with pericardial effusions
D cardiac tamponade is usually associated with pulmonary oedema
E pericardial paracentesis is likely to be necessary if the JVP and the pulse rate both rise with expiration

100
Given the development of acute pericarditis in a 20 year old woman, the following disorders should be excluded
A Hodgkin's disease
B systemic lupus erythematosus
C Coxsackie A virus infection
D acute rheumatic fever
E rubella virus infection

101
The following statements about constrictive pericarditis are true
A breathlessness is characteristically severe
B ascites and hepatomegaly are rarely present at onset
C there is usually a previous history of TB or haemopericardium
D tachycardia, cardiomegaly and a third heart sound are present
E the JVP is markedly elevated with a steep 'y' descent

102
Central cyanosis in infancy is an expected finding in the following congenital heart diseases
A persistent ductus arteriosus
B transposition of the great arteries
C coarctation of the aorta
D Fallot's tetralogy
E atrial septal defect

103
The following statements about persistent ductus arteriosus are true
A foetal blood passes from the aorta to the pulmonary artery
B the disorder is much commoner in male infants
C a systolic murmur is usually present around the scapulae
D shunt reversal is indicated by cyanosis of the lower limbs
E surgical ligation is inadvisable if central cyanosis is present

Answers
98 A B C D E
99 none
100 A B D

101 C E
102 B D
103 D E

104
Typical clinical features of coarctation of the aorta include
A an association with bicuspid aortic valve
B cardiac failure developing in male adolescents
C palpable collateral arteries around the scapulae
D rib-notching on chest x-ray associated with weak femoral pulses
E continuous murmur at the left upper sternal edge associated with a heaving and displaced apex beat

105
In atrial septal defect
A there is a male preponderance
B the initial shunt is right to left
C splitting of the second heart sound increases in expiration
D a tricuspid systolic flow murmur is usually present
E surgery should be deferred until shunt reversal occurs

106
In small ventricular septal defects
A a mid-systolic murmur is maximal at the left sternal edge
B the heart is usually enlarged and CRBBB on ECG is often present
C there is a risk of infective endocarditis
D most small VSDs require surgical repair before adolescence
E most patients are asymptomatic

107
In right to left shunt reversal (Eisenmenger's syndrome) of congenital heart disease
A pulmonary arterial hypertension is usually present
B prompt closure of the ASD or VSD produces symptomatic relief
C recurrent respiratory infections are characteristically present
D most patients have central cyanosis and finger clubbing
E shunt murmurs are prominent when polycythaemia is severe

108
In Fallot's tetralogy
A pulmonary and aortic stenosis are combined with a VSD
B finger clubbing and central cyanosis are present from birth
C the second heart sound is loud and widely split on inspiration
D the chest X-ray and ECG are typically abnormal
E beta blockade is useful in the emergency treatment of cyanotic spells prior to surgical correction

109
Cardiovascular changes in normal pregnancy include
A cardiac output increases by 150% by 12 weeks
B tachycardia, elevated JVP and third heart sound
C reduction in systemic diastolic pressure
D pulmonary systolic murmur
E reduced blood coagulability post partum

Answers
104 A C D
105 none
106 C E

107 A C D
108 D E
109 B C D

110
In a pregnant woman with
A mitral stenosis, termination is advisable
B central cyanosis and a VSD, maternal mortality is about 33%
C a ligated ductus arteriosus, pregnancy should be uncomplicated
D a prosthetic heart valve, warfarin therapy should be continued
E asymptomatic mitral stenosis at 24 weeks, an uncomplicated delivery is likely

111
Recognised causes of deep vein thrombosis (DVT) include
A pregnancy and oestrogen therapy
B polycythaemia
C prolonged travelling
D cardiac failure
E carcinomatosis

112
The clinical features suggesting the presence of DVT include
A cold, painful, blue limb with altered sensation
B prominent superficial veins disappearing on limb elevation
C warm, painless, oedematous, white limb
D calf tenderness and fever
E syncopal episode during defaecation

113
The following statements about intermittent claudication due to atherosclerosis are true
A the pain is typically relieved by rest and elevation of the leg
B the skin, hair and nail changes are characteristic of ischaemia
C normal peripheral pulses suggest anaemia or beta blocker therapy
D absence of arterial bruits is common when systemic BP is normal
E leg elevation produces blanching which, after placing the leg in a dependent position, is followed by flushing and venous filling

114
Raynaud's phenomenon is a recognised association of
A thromboangiitis obliterans (Buerger's disease)
B cryoglobulinaemia
C progressive systemic sclerosis
D vibration trauma
E giant cell arteritis

115
Arterial embolism is a recognised complication of
A left atrial myxoma
B atrial septal defect
C myocardial infarction
D infective endocarditis
E persistent ductus arteriosus

116
Clinical features compatible with acute arterial embolism include
A warm, painful, swollen leg
B left pleuritic chest pain
C painful, cold, leg with altered sensation
D recent onset of atrial fibrillation
E onset of stroke after myocardial infarction

117
The risk of dissecting aortic aneurysm is increased in
A Marfan's syndrome
B coarctation of the aorta
C pregnancy
D Takayasu disease
E syphilitic aortitis

118
Characteristic features of dissecting aortic aneurysm include
A haemopericardium
B acute flaccid paraparesis
C interscapular back pain
D cardiogenic shock
E normal peripheral pulses

Answers
110 B C
111 A B C D E
112 C D E
113 C E

114 A B C D
115 A B C D
116 B C D E
117 A B C D E
118 A B C

119
Typical features of polyarteritis nodosa include
A preponderance in elderly females
B involvement of the smaller arterioles
C abdominal pain and weight loss
D angina and mononeuritis multiplex
E hypertension and haematuria

120
Typical laboratory findings in polyarteritis nodosa include
A peripheral blood lymphocytosis
B elevated plasma LDH and ALT concentrations
C microscopic haematuria and red cell casts
D transient chest X-ray opacities
E restrictive pattern of pulmonary function tests

121
Clinical features of giant cell arteritis include
A proximal muscle stiffness and tenderness
B occipital or temporal headache with scalp tenderness
C jaw claudication and uniocular blindness
D weight loss, night sweats and fever
E dramatic response to prednisolone 60 mg daily

Answers
119 C D E
120 B C D

121 A B C D E

Diseases of the respiratory system

1
The following statements about acute respiratory illness are characteristic
A pneumococcal pneumonia — pleural pain precedes fever
B viral pneumonia — cough precedes other symptoms
C pulmonary TB — physical signs in the chest are prominent
D atypical pneumonia — physical signs are at variance with symptoms
E pulmonary infarct — the absence of symptoms excludes the diagnosis

2
Chest pain and cough are typically both present in
A chronic bronchitis
B acute tracheitis
C acute asthma
D pneumococcal pneumonia
E pulmonary infarction

3
Cough is an expected feature of
A maxillary sinusitis
B acute bronchiolitis
C fibrosing alveolitis
D acute pharyngitis
E miliary tuberculosis

4
The following sputum characteristics are associated with
A rusty-coloured — staphylococcal pneumonia
B watery consistency — chronic asthma
C foul-smelling — lung abscess
D pink and frothy — pulmonary oedema
E black — chronic bronchitis

5
Sputum consisting only of blood is an expected finding in
A pulmonary infarction
B bronchiectasis
C pulmonary TB
D acute asthma
E aortic stenosis

6
Pleuritic chest pain is a characteristic feature of
A splenic infarction
B hepatic infarction
C pneumothorax
D pericarditis
E rib fracture

7
The following features are typical of wheeze
A induced by exertion even if absent at rest
B louder in inspiration rather than expiration
C pitch is inversely related to the airway diameter
D nocturnal occurrence suggests cardiac failure
E induced by coughing in chronic bronchitis more than asthma

8
Persistent nasal obstruction is a recognised feature of
A diphtheria
B impacted foreign body
C allergic rhinitis
D adenoidal enlargement
E nasal septal deformity

Answers
1 D
2 B D
3 B C D
4 C D

5 A B C
6 A B C D E
7 A C
8 B C D E

9
Expected features of acute laryngitis include
A haemoptysis
B hoarseness
C stridor
D 'barking' cough
E high-pitched wheeze

10
Typical features of stridor include
A accentuation by coughing
B louder on expiration than inspiration
C higher pitch in tracheal than laryngeal obstruction
D usually accompanied by breathlessness
E early onset of central cyanosis

11
Central cyanosis is an expected finding in
A SVC obstruction
B fibrosing alveolitis
C polycythaemia
D hypothermia
E chronic bronchitis

12
Clinical features of finger clubbing include
A increased nail curvature
B nail base telangiectasia
C nail base skin oedema
D nail base fluctuation
E finger pulp swelling

13
Finger clubbing is a typical finding in
A chronic bronchitis
B bronchiectasis
C primary biliary cirrhosis
D fibrosing alveolitis
E ventricular septal defect

14
Tracheal deviation to the right is an expected finding in
A right main bronchus occlusion
B right lower lobe pneumonia
C right pleural effusion
D right upper lobe fibrosis
E right tension pneumothorax

15
Hyperinflation of the chest is suggested by
A pectus excavatum
B AP diameter = lateral diameter
C increased crico-sternal distance
D intercostal muscle indrawing
E maximum chest expansion = 5 cm

16
An increased AP chest diameter is a typical finding in
A chronic bronchitis
B pectus carinatum
C thoracoplasty
D thoracic kyphoscoliosis
E pneumothorax

Answers
9 B C D
10 A D
11 B C
12 A C D E

13 B C D
14 A D
15 B D
16 A B D

17
Reduced maximum chest expansion is a recognised feature of
A normal pregnancy
B ankylosing spondylitis
C primary pulmonary hypertension
D fibrosing alveolitis
E pulmonary emphysema

18
Thoracic rather than abdominal respiratory movements typify
A ascites
B pleurisy
C ankylosing spondylitis
D normal adult males
E peritonitis

19
Hyperpnoea is a typical feature of
A emphysema
B uraemia
C aspirin poisoning
D diabetic ketoacidosis
E ankylosing spondylitis

20
Typical chest findings in a large right pleural effusion include
A normal chest expansion
B dull percussion note
C absent breath sounds
D decreased vocal resonance
E pleural friction rub

21
Typical chest findings in right lower lobe consolidation include
A decreased chest expansion
B dull percussion note
C decreased breath sounds
D increased vocal resonance
E rhonchi and crepitations

22
Typical chest findings in right lower lobe collapse include
A decreased chest expansion
B stony dull percussion note
C bronchial breath sounds
D decreased vocal resonance
E crepitations

23
Typical chest findings in a large right pneumothorax include
A decreased chest expansion
B normal percussion note
C increased breath sounds
D increased vocal resonance
E absence of added sounds

24
The characteristics of bronchial breath sounds include
A increased loudness of both inspiratory and expiratory sounds
B absence of an audible gap between inspiration and expiration
C harsh blowing quality of the expiratory sound alone
D inspiratory sound audibly more prolonged than expiratory sound
E increased vocal resonance is always present

Answers
17 B D E
18 A E
19 B C D
20 C D

21 A B D
22 A D
23 A B E
24 A E

25
Vocal resonance is typically increased in
A bronchial carcinoma
B fibrosing alveolitis
C empyema thoracis
D primary pulmonary TB
E haemopneumothorax

26
Breath sounds are typically diminished or absent in
A pneumothorax
B pleural effusion
C bronchiectasis
D consolidation due to pneumonia
E collapse due to bronchial obstruction

27
Coughing usually modifies the following added sounds
A pleural friction rub due to pneumonia
B crepitations due to pulmonary oedema
C crepitations due to pneumonia
D crepitations due to fibrosing alveolitis
E rhonchus due to malignant bronchial obstruction

28
The following disorders usually present with acute dyspnoea and chest pain
A bronchial asthma
B chronic bronchitis
C myocardial infarction
D pulmonary embolism
E pneumothorax

29
In a patient with recurrent paroxysmal nocturnal dyspnoea, the following features favour asthma rather than cardiac failure
A end-inspiratory crepitations
B central cyanosis without peripheral cyanosis
C pulsus paradoxus and sinus arrhythmia
D elevated jugular venous pressure
E expiratory rhonchi without other signs

30
Dyspnoea is usually due to decreased pulmonary compliance in
A pulmonary embolism
B ankylosing spondylitis
C chronic bronchitis and emphysema
D pneumococcal pneumonia
E pulmonary oedema

31
Orthopnoea is an expected finding in
A chronic anaemia
B chronic bronchitis and emphysema
C left ventricular failure
D spontaneous pneumothorax
E pulmonary embolism

32
In the normal adult
A the trachea bifurcates at the level of the suprasternal notch
B the left main bronchus is more vertical than the right
C the right lung usually has ten bronchopulmonary segments
D the oblique fissure extends from the thoracic vertebral level T3
E pulmonary surfactant is secreted by Type I pneumocytes

Answers
25 B
26 A B E
27 B C
28 C D E

29 B C E
30 D E
31 B C
32 C D

33
The following statements about pulmonary anatomy are true
A the middle lobe lies posteror to the right upper lobe
B the left upper lobe lies anterior to the left lower lobe
C the ciliated epithelium extends down to the terminal bronchioles
D the parietal and visceral pleura are continuous at the hilum
E the transverse fissure separates the right middle lobe from the right lower lobe

34
In the normal resting adult
A pulmonary ventilation is 10 litres per minute
B alveolar ventilation is 5 litres per minute
C pulmonary blood flow is 10 litres per minute
D the PaO_2 is 11–13 kPa and $PaCO_2$ is 4.8–6.0 kPa
E the pulmonary blood carries 250 ml/min (11 mmol) of oxygen to the tissues and excretes 200 ml/min (9 mmol) of carbon dioxide

35
The metabolic cost of ventilation attributable to elastic work (work done against elastic resistance) is increased by
A ankylosing spondylitis
B chronic bronchitis
C bronchial asthma
D pulmonary oedema
E obstruction of a main bronchus

36
In the central control of breathing
A fever reduces the sensitivity of the respiratory centre
B only central chemoreceptors are sensitive to arterial PCO_2
C peripheral chemoreceptors are sensitive only to arterial PO_2
D chronic alveolar hypoventilation decreases sensitivity to arterial PCO_2
E limb, chest wall and pulmonary stretch receptors stimulate ventilation during exercise

37
Alveolar hypoventilation is typically associated with
A pulmonary embolism
B severe chest wall deformity
C salicylate intoxication
D pulmonary fibrosis
E severe chronic bronchitis

38
The following disorders are associated with decreased alveolar ventilation and perfusion (V/Q) ratios
A chronic bronchitis
B pulmonary embolism
C atrial septal defect
D lobar pneumonia
E kyphoscoliosis

39
The gas transfer factor or diffusion capacity is
A the diffusion rate of oxygen across the alveolar membrane
B decreased in emphysema
C independent of changes in the V/Q ratio
D decreased in fibrosing alveolitis
E decreased by about 50% following pneumonectomy

Answers
33 B C D
34 B D E
35 A D

36 D E
37 B E
38 A D E
39 B D

40
The following statements about pulmonary function tests are true
A over 80% of vital capacity can normally be expelled in 1 second
B forced expiratory times > 3 seconds indicate FEV/FVC ratios < 50%
C residual volume is increased in chronic bronchitis and emphysema
D the FEV/FVC ratio is usually normal in ankylosing spondylitis
E peak expiratory flow rates provide a useful index of the severity of restrictive ventilatory defects

41
Typical clinical features of chronic hypercapnia include
A retinal venous distension
B drowsiness
C cold clammy skin
D headache
E muscle twitching

42
The following disorders characteristically produce type I respiratory failure
A kyphoscoliosis
B Guillain–Barre polyneuropathy
C adult respiratory distress syndrome
D extrinsic allergic alveolitis
E emphysema

43
The following disorders characteristically produce type II respiratory failure
A chronic bronchitis
B poliomyelitis
C pulmonary embolism
D fibrosing alveolitis
E bronchial asthma

44
The following statements about oxygen therapy are true
A at sea level, the pressure of oxygen in inspired air is 20 kPa
B normal arterial blood contains 200 ml (9 mmol) of oxygen/litre
C dissolved oxygen contributes to tissue oxygenation in anaemia
D oxygen toxicity in adults can produce retrolental fibroplasia
E central cyanosis unresponsive to 100% oxygen in inspired air indicates right-to-left shunting of > 20% of cardiac output

45
In the delivery of oxygen therapy, the following statements are true
A MC mask: inspired oxygen concentration = 80% at 8 L/min
B Ventimask: prevention of the rebreathing of carbon dioxide
C nasal cannulae: inspired oxygen concentration = 30% at 2 L/min
D Ventimask: oxygen should be humidified by passage through water
E written prescription of both the method of delivery and the flow rate are essential

46
Mechanical ventilation (IPPV) is usually indicated when acute type II respiratory failure is the result of
A acute opiate intoxication
B acute bronchial asthma
C severe pneumonia complicating chronic bronchitis
D flail chest injury following a road traffic accident
E pulmonary oedema associated with cardiogenic shock

Answers
40 C D
41 A B D E
42 C D E
43 A B

44 A B C E
45 B C E
46 B C D

47
In the treatment of chronic bronchitis associated with chronic type II respiratory failure
A oxygen should be given using an MC mask at 2 L/min
B nebulised doxapram improves small airways obstruction
C cough disturbing sleep should be treated with pholcodeine
D corticosteroid therapy is usually contraindicated
E continuous oxygen therapy can reduce pulmonary hypertension

48
Adult respiratory distress syndrome is associated with
A alveolar oedema with a protein content 20 g/L
B hypoxaemia and systemic hypotension
C severe dyspnoea with rhonchi rather than crepitations
D widespread 'fluffy' or 'soft' opacification on chest X-ray
E thrombocytopenia and disseminated intravascular coagulation

49
The following acute respiratory tract disorders are usually attributable to the viral infections listed below
A laryngotracheobronchitis (croup) — Coxsackie A virus
B epiglottitis — rhinoviruses
C bronchiolitis — respiratory syncytial virus
D viral pneumonia — enteroviruses
E pharyngoconjunctival fever — echoviruses

50
Influenza A and B viral infections are associated with
A short-lived type-specific immunity following infection
B an incubation period of 7–10 days
C leucopenia
D acute tracheobronchitis
E staphylococcal bronchopneumonia

51
Typical clinical features of acute tracheobronchitis include
A an irritating unproductive cough at onset
B superinfection with *Staphylococcus aureus*
C retrosternal chest pain
D pyrexia and neutrophil leucocytosis
E crepitations rather than rhonchi on auscultation

52
Characteristic features of pneumococcal pneumonia include
A sudden onset of rigors and pleuritic pain
B peak frequency in childhood and old age
C lobar collapse and diminished breath sounds
D bacteraemia and neutrophil leucocytosis
E herpes labialis

53
Recognised complications of pneumococcal pneumonia include
A bronchial carcinoma
B pericarditis
C peripheral circulatory failure
D pleural effusion and empyema
E subphrenic abscess

54
Typical features of staphylococcal pneumonia include
A an illness clinically indistinguishable from pneumococcal pneumonia
B multiple lung abscesses which persist as thin-walled cysts
C association with influenza A infection
D staphylococcal sepsis elsewhere in the body
E penicillin-resistance

Answers
47 E
48 B D E
49 C E
50 A C D E

51 A C D
52 A D E
53 B C D
54 A B C D E

55
Typical features of *Klebsiella pneumonia* include
A upper lobe collapse on chest X-ray
B severe systemic disturbance and high mortality
C copious chocolate-coloured sputum
D organisms resistant to chloramphenicol and gentamycin
E occurrence in previously healthy individuals

56
Recognised features of *Mycoplasmal pneumonia* include
A institutional outbreaks in young adults
B haemolytic anaemia and cold agglutinins in the serum
C fever and malaise preceding respiratory symptoms by several days
D inconspicuous physical signs in the chest
E response to tetracycline or erythromycin therapy

57
Typical features of *Legionella pneumonia* include
A oro-faecal spread of infection
B vomiting and diarrhoea
C hyponatraemia and confusion
D inconspicuous physical signs in the chest
E response to rifampicin and/or erythromycin therapy

58
Pneumonia due to infections other than *Streptococcus pneumoniae* are more likely if the clinical features include
A respiratory symptoms preceding systemic upset by several days
B chest signs at variance with the chest X-ray appearances
C the development of a pleural effusion
D the absence of a neutrophil leucocytosis
E palpable splenomegaly and proteinuria

59
Pneumonia in immunocompromised individuals due to opportunistic infections is best treated with the following drug regimes
A *Pneumocystis carinii* — co-trimoxazole
B *Pseudomonas aeruginosa* — azlocillin or ciprofloxacin
C cytomegalovirus — ganciclovir
D *Herpes simplex* — acyclovir
E respiratory syncytial virus — tribavirin

60
Typical features of acute bronchopneumonia include
A occurrence in middle-aged adults
B occurrence after debilitating illness and influenza
C absence of a neutrophil leucocytosis
D acute onset with pleuritic chest pain
E bronchiectasis and fibrosis are recognised complications

61
The following statements about aspiration pneumonias are true
A bronchiectasis is a recognised complication
B chest X-ray abnormalities are typically bilateral
C lobar collapse predisposes to the development of lung abscess
D systemic upset is usually marked
E clinical and radiological resolution are generally rapid

62
The clinical features of suppurative pneumonia and lung abscess include
A prior pulmonary infarction
B the presence of an inhaled foreign body
C rigors and pleuritic chest pain
D bronchial breathing if attributable to an obstructing carcinoma
E radiological features of cavitation

Answers
55 B C
56 A B C D E
57 B C D E
58 B D E

59 A B C D E
60 B E
61 A C E
62 A B C E

63
Post-primary tuberculosis in Britain is associated with
A occurrence in childhood rather than old age
B an increased prevalence in diabetic patients
C human rather than bovine strains of mycobacteriae
D alcohol abuse and malnutrition
E air-borne reinfection rather than reactivation of infection

64
Typical features of primary tuberculosis include
A a sustained pyrexial illness
B caseation within the regional lymph nodes
C bilateral hilar lymphadenopathy on chest X-ray
D erythema nodosum
E pleural effusion with a negative tuberculin skin test

65
Recognised features of miliary tuberculosis include
A severe systemic upset with fever in childhood
B blood dyscrasias and hepatosplenomegaly
C normal chest X-ray and negative tuberculin test
D inconspicuous physical signs in the chest
E characteristic granulomata on liver and bone biopsy

66
Typical features of post-primary tuberculosis include
A purulent sputum negative for TB on microscopy
B bilateral upper lobe opacities on chest X-ray
C conspicuous physical signs in the chest
D epididymitis and ureteric obstruction
E ischiorectal abscess and intestinal obstruction

67
Recognised complications of post-primary tuberculosis include
A aspergilloma
B amyloidosis
C miliary tuberculosis
D bronchiectasis
E paraplegia

68
The following statements about tuberculin Tine testing are true
A false positives are common in sarcoidosis and acute exanthemata
B the skin reaction is best assessed 3 days after innoculation
C tuberculin-positive family contacts do not require BCG vaccination
D grade III and IV reactions are characterised by 4 discrete papules
E tuberculin-positive children are immune to tuberculosis

69
In the treatment of post-primary pulmonary tuberculosis
A combination drug therapy is always indicated
B sputum culture for TB often remains positive for at least 3 months
C at least 12 months daily therapy is required for 100% effectiveness
D isoniazid and pyrazinamide do not cross the blood-brain barrier
E treatment failure is invariably due to multiple drug resistance

70
Recognised adverse reactions to anti-tuberculous drugs include
A streptomycin — renal failure
B isoniazid — hypothyroidism
C rifampicin — optic neuritis
D pyrazinamide — hepatitis
E ethambutol — vestibular neuronitis

Answers
63 B C D
64 B D
65 A B C D E
66 B D E

67 A B C D E
68 B C
69 A
70 D

71
Prophylactic anti-tuberculous drug therapy should be administered to the following tuberculin-positive individuals
A type I insulin-dependent diabetics
B patients receiving long-term immunosuppressant drug therapy
C HIV antibody positive subjects
D children aged < 3 years who have not received BCG vaccine
E adults who have recently become tuberculin-positive

72
Pulmonary infection with *Aspergillus fumigatus* is a recognised cause of the following
A bullous emphysema
B mycetoma
C necrotising pneumonitis
D bronchopulmonary eosinophilia
E extrinsic allergic alveolitis

73
Typical features of seasonal allergic rhinitis include
A cell-mediated delayed hypersensitivity response to pollens
B sneezing and lachrimation
C purulent nasal discharge
D positive skin sensitivity tests
E response to ipratropium nasal spray

74
Typical features of early onset bronchial asthma include
A individuals are usually atopic
B a single allergen can often be identified
C paroxysmal expiratory wheeze and dyspnoea
D a strong family history of allergic disorders
E aspergillus fumigatus is usually present in the sputum

75
Typical features of late onset bronchial asthma include
A association with nasal polyps
B multiple allergens can often be identified
C exposure to aspirin and certain chemicals can induce attacks
D asthma is more often chronic than episodic
E serum IgE concentrations are often normal

76
Features indicative of severe acute asthma include
A pulse rate = 120 per minute
B peak expiratory flow rate = 350 L per minute
C pulsus paradoxus = 30 mm Hg
D arterial PaO_2 = 10 kPa
E arterial $PaCO_2$ = 6 kPa

77
The initial management of severe acute asthma should include
A 28% oxygen using a Ventimask
B salbutamol 2.5 mg i.v. or 5 mg by inhalation
C ampicillin 500 mg i.v. and cromoglycate 10 mg by inhalation
D hydrocortisone 200 mg i.v. and prednisolone 40 mg orally
E arterial blood gas analysis and chest X-ray

78
The typical features of asthmatic pulmonary eosinophilia include
A immediate hypersensitivity and immune complex reactions
B positive skin and serum tests for *Aspergillus fumigatus*
C isolation of *Aspergillus clavatus* in the sputum
D recurrent upper lobe collapse
E chronic asthma and bronchiectasis

Answers
71 B C D E
72 B C D
73 B D E
74 A C D

75 A C D E
76 A C E
77 B D E
78 A B D E

79
Characteristic features of pulmonary eosinophilia include
A an association with ascariasis and microfilariasis
B eosinophilic pneumonia without peripheral blood eosinophilia
C prominent asthmatic features
D induction by exposure to sulphonamide drugs
E lower lobar collapse on chest X-ray

80
Clinical features compatible with a diagnosis of extrinsic allergic alveolitis include
A expiratory rhonchi and sputum eosinophilia
B dry cough, dyspnoea and pyrexia
C end-inspiratory crepitations
D FEV_1/FVC ratio = 60%
E positive serum precipitin test

81
Pathognomonic features of chronic bronchitis include
A decreased residual volume
B recurrent acute bronchitis
C decreased mucus secretion
D increased FEV_1/FVC ratio
E cough and breathlessness for more than 2 months every year

82
Recognised features of pulmonary emphysema include
A absence of airways obstruction if chronic bronchitis is absent
B central cyanosis as an early manifestation
C reduced carbon monoxide transfer factor
D dyspnoea more prominent than in chronic bronchitis
E alpha$_1$-antitrypsin deficiency in young adults

83
Characteristic findings in pulmonary emphysema during inspiration include
A filling of the internal jugular veins
B tracheal descent
C indrawing of the intercostal muscles
D contraction of the scalene muscles
E widespread rhonchi

84
Typical findings on the chest X-ray in chronic bronchitis and emphysema include
A prominent pulmonary arteries at the hila
B low flat diaphragms
C prominent peripheral vascular markings
D upper lobe pulmonary venous congestion
E Kerley A lines and cardiomegaly

85
Recognised causes of bronchiectasis include
A primary hypogammaglobulinaemia
B an inhaled foreign body
C cystic fibrosis
D asthmatic pulmonary eosinophilia
E sarcoidosis

86
Typical clinical features of bronchiectasis include
A chronic cough with scanty sputum volumes
B recurrent pleurisy
C haemoptysis
D empyema thoracis
E crepitations on auscultation

Answers
79 A D
80 B C E
81 none
82 C D E

83 B C D
84 A B
85 A B C D
86 B C D E

87
In the treatment of bronchiectasis
A postural drainage is best undertaken for 10 minutes twice daily
B failure of medical therapy is a clear indication for surgery
C antibiotic therapy is indicated if sputum purulence persists
D bronchography is required before surgery is undertaken
E pulmonary emphysema is a contraindication to surgery

88
The following statements about bronchial obstruction are true
A emphysema develops in the presence of partial obstruction
B mediastinal displacement is always towards the affected side
C infection is inevitable especially in partial obstruction
D a collapsed right middle lobe is best detected radiologically
E inhaled foreign bodies usually lodge in the left main bronchus

89
Typical features of bronchial adenoma include
A occurrence in elderly females
B carcinoid syndrome if liver metastases are present
C recurrent haemoptysis
D lobar emphysema
E recurrent pneumonia

90
The following statements about bronchial carcinoma are true
A accounts for 10% of all male deaths from cancer
B typically presents with massive haemoptysis
C the histology in 50% is adenocarcinoma
D is associated with asbestos exposure
E is 40 times more common in smokers than non-smokers

91
Bronchial carcinoma
A is surgically resectable in approximately 30%
B can be excluded if the chest X-ray is normal
C has a 50% 5 year survival after surgical resection
D can only be diagnosed reliably by bronchoscopy
E associated with finger clubbing suggests a small cell histology

92
Non-metastatic manifestations of bronchial carcinoma include
A cerebellar degeneration
B myasthenia
C gynaecomastia
D polyneuropathy
E dermatomyositis

93
Typical presentations of small cell bronchial carcinoma include
A nephrotic syndrome
B inappropriate ADH secretion
C ectopic ACTH secretion
D ectopic parathyroid hormone secretion
E hypertrophic pulmonary osteoarthropathy

94
Typical features of cryptogenic fibrosing alveolitis include
A hypercapnic respiratory failure
B positive antinuclear and rheumatoid factors
C finger clubbing
D recurrent wheeze and haemoptysis
E increased neutrophil and eosinophil count in bronchial washings

---

Answers
87 A D E
88 A C D
89 B C D E
90 D E

91 none
92 A B C D E
93 A B C
94 B C E

95
In coal-worker's pneumoconiosis
A the disease usually progresses despite avoidance of coal dust
B certification for compensation depends upon the clinical features
C upper lobe opacities suggest progressive massive fibrosis
D accompanying chronic bronchitis is not due to coal dust exposure
E physical findings are often in evidence

96
Typical findings in silicosis include
A chest X-ray abnormalities similar to those found in coal-workers
B 'egg-shell' calcification of the hilar lymph nodes
C progression of the disease arrested when dust exposure ceases
D fibrotic peripheral nodules in patients with rheumatoid disease
E occupational history of coal, tin and mineral mining

97
The following statements about asbestos-related disease are true
A pleural plaques usually progress to become mesotheliomas
B benign pleural effusions are never blood-stained
C finger clubbing and basal crepitations suggest pulmonary asbestosis
D the FEV_1/FVC ratio is typically decreased
E mesothelioma is best diagnosed at thoracotomy

98
Occupational exposure to the following antigens produce pulmonary disorders attributable to an extrinsic allergic alveolitis
A cotton dust — bagassosis
B mouldy hay — farmer's lung
C tin dioxide — siderosis
D avian protein — bird fancier's lung
E mouldy sugar cane — bysinnosis

99
The following statements about sarcoidosis are true
A pulmonary lesions characteristically cavitate
B the tuberculin tine test is usually positive
C erythema marginatum is the typical skin lesion
D spontaneous resolution is unusual
E hypercalcaemia suggests skeletal involvement

100
Typical features of subacute sarcoidosis include
A hilar lymphadenopathy on chest X-ray
B cranial neuropathies
C conjunctivitis
D erosive polyarthritis
E swollen parotid glands

101
The development of a pleural effusion with a protein content of 50 G per litre would be compatible with
A congestive cardiac failure
B pulmonary infarction
C subphrenic abscess
D pneumonia
E nephrotic syndrome

102
In a patient with a symptomatic pleural effusion
A physical signs in the chest are invariably present
B pleural biopsy should be avoided given a protein content of 50 G/L
C TB can be excluded if the chest X-ray is otherwise normal
D lymphocytosis in the pleural fluid is pathognomonic of pleural TB
E milky pleural fluid suggests thoracic duct obstruction

Answers

95 C D
96 A B D E
97 C
98 B D

99 none
100 A B E
101 B C D
102 A E

103
Typical features of an empyema thoracis include
A bilateral effusions on chest X-ray
B a fluid level on chest X-ray suggests a bronchopleural fistula
C persistent pyrexia despite antibiotic therapy
D recent abdominal surgery
E bacteriological culture of the organism despite antibiotic therapy

104
The following statements about spontaneous pneumothorax are true
A breathlessness and pleuritic chest pain are usually present
B bronchial breathing is audible over the affected hemithorax
C absent peripheral lung markings on chest X-ray suggests tension
D surgical referral is required if there is a bronchopleural fistula
E pleurodesis should be considered for recurrent pneumothoraces

Answers
103 B C D

104 A D E

Diseases of the alimentary tract and pancreas

1

The following statements about alimentary symptoms are true

A waterbrash is the reflux of gastric acid

B globus is a typical feature of bulbar palsy

C heartburn rarely occurs without overt oesophagitis

D odynophagia usually indicates the presence of oesophagitis

E vomiting without preceding nausea is typical of migraine

2

The following symptoms invariably indicate a structural abnormality of the alimentary tract

A dysphagia localised to the xiphisternum

B abdominal distension and borborygmi

C heartburn and acid regurgitation

D epigastric fullness after meals

E epigastric pain with rebound tenderness

3

The pain associated with peptic oesophagitis

A responds poorly to antacid therapy

B is aggravated by swallowing hot liquids

C is easily distinguishable from ischaemic chest pain

D is aggravated by bending and relieved by standing

E can be differentiated from duodenal ulcer dyspepsia by the fact that nocturnal pain is exceptional in oesophagitis

4

Abdominal pain is a characteristic feature of

A intestinal spirochaetosis

B lead poisoning

C acute intermittent porphyria

D diabetic ketoacidosis

E tricyclic antidepressant poisoning

5

Typical features of peptic ulcer dyspepsia include

A sharp stabbing epigastric pain

B well-localised pain relieved by vomiting

C pain-free remissions lasting many weeks

D nausea and epigastric pain relieved by belching

E nocturnal pain causing frequent night waking

6

Typical features of biliary colic include

A pain radiating to the right shoulder tip or scapula

B colicky pain recurring every 2–5 minutes

C nausea and vomiting

D restlessness and sweating

E pain relieved by bland food

7

Typical features of acute pancreatitis include

A colicky pain recurring every 2–5 minutes

B pain lessened by sitting forwards

C hyperactive loud bowel sounds

D nausea and vomiting

E back pain radiating to the groins

Answers

1 D

2 A E

3 B D

4 B C D

5 B C E

6 A C D

7 B D

8
Typical features of renal colic include
A nausea and vomiting
B pain lessened by lying still
C dysuria and pneumaturia
D pain lasting 4–24 hours continuously
E prompt relief with intravenous atropine therapy

9
The following structures are often palpable in the normal abdomen
A right kidney
B spleen
C left kidney
D liver
E pancreas

10
On abdominal palpation
A renal tenderness is typically most marked anteriorly
B the kidneys descend on inspiration
C splenic enlargement is characterised by a palpably notched edge
D a palpable sigmoid colon is pathological
E on a jaundiced patient gallbladder enlargement suggests stones in the common bile duct

11
On percussion of the abdomen
A dullness in the flanks is usually pathological
B central dullness suggests an enlarged pelvic organ
C the liver size is likely to be overestimated
D shifting dullness is typical of an ovarian cyst
E resonance over a left hypochondrial mass suggests splenomegaly

12
During digital examination of the rectum
A an empty rectum is an expected finding in healthy subjects
B seminal vesicles are often palpable in the normal male
C haemorrhoids are impalpable unless thrombosed
D prostatic palpation often induces the desire to micturate
E an anterior pelvic mass palpable during the menses is likely to be due to the presence of a vaginal tampon

13
In a patient with severe acute abdominal pain
A analgesics should be withheld pending confirmation of the diagnosis
B visible peristalsis suggests intestinal obstruction
C peritonitis is characterised by hyperactive loud bowel sounds
D lower lobe pneumonia should be considered among possible diagnoses
E perforation is likely if vomiting and restlessness are marked

14
In the neuroendocrinal control of the alimentary tract
A neural control is mediated by mucosal hormone secretion
B the initial release of gastrin occurs in response to food intake
C sympathetic nerve fibres run in the splanchnic nerves
D parasympathetic nerves mediate the inhibition of hormone secretion
E exocrine pancreatic secretion is controlled solely by hormonal factors

Answers
  8 A D
  9 A D
10 B C
11 B

12 A C D E
13 B D
14 A C

15
The following statements about gastrointestinal motility are true
A the lower oesophageal sphincter is controlled solely by neural factors
B the upper oesophageal sphincter is relaxed except during swallowing
C initial gastric relaxation on eating is vagally mediated
D normally, 50% of gastric solids are emptied within 30 minutes of ingestion
E vagotomy delays gastric emptying of liquids more than solids

16
In the control of the motility of the alimentary tract
A the myenteric plexus determines the local response to the 'slow wave'
B the 'slow wave' frequency is greater in the ileum than the duodenum
C colonic motility is inhibited following food ingestion
D propulsion of colonic contents is inhibited by segmentation
E increased colonic motility is a typical finding in diarrhoea

17
The following statements about the enteric hormonal control of alimentary secretions are true
A gastrin secretion is inhibited by a rise in intragastric pH
B secretin and cholecystokinin stimulate gastric acid secretion
C secretin stimulates pancreatic enzyme secretion
D cholecystokinin stimulates pancreatic bicarbonate secretion
E somatostatin increases hormonal and gastrointestinal secretions

18
In the normal alimentary tract
A the small bowel surface epithelium is replaced every 48 hours
B secretory IgA protects the gut from bacterial invasion
C fat soluble drugs and vitamins are transported via the lymphatics
D folic acid is chiefly absorbed in the distal jejunum and ileum
E approximately 1.5 L of fluid passes into the caecum daily

19
The following statements about human dentition are true
A adults should normally have 32 teeth
B all but the third molars should have erupted by the age of 12
C bright white teeth suggest fluorosis in childhood
D juvenile hypoparathyroidism results in hypoplastic teeth
E tetracycline therapy in childhood produces yellowing of the teeth

20
The following statements about diseases of the mouth are true
A aphthous ulcers are usually due to herpes simplex infection
B aphthous ulcers are a typical feature in gluten enteropathy
C hairy leucoplakia is pathognomonic of HIV infection
D pain in the tongue aggravated by hot liquids suggests leukoplakia
E bluish discoloration of the gums is typical of chronic lead poisoning

21
Recognised causes of stomatitis include
A lichen planus
B psoriasis
C erythema multiforme
D herpes simplex
E candidiasis

Answers
15 C D
16 A D
17 none

18 A B C E
19 B D E
20 B C
21 A C D E

22
The following statements about gingivitis are true
A phenytoin produces gum hypertrophy
B Vincent's angina is caused by Coxsackie A infection
C scurvy is a particularly unlikely cause in an edentulous patient
D syphilis should be considered if the condition is painful
E tetracycline is the therapy of choice if ulceration is present

23
Vomiting in the morning is a typical feature of
A pyloric obstruction
B alcohol abuse
C raised intracranial pressure
D gallstones
E pregnancy

24
Recognised causes of dysphagia include
A iron deficiency anaemia
B pharyngeal pouch
C Barrett's oesophagus
D myasthenia gravis
E African trypanosomiasis

25
The following statements about pharyngeal pouch are true
A affected patients should sleep in a semi-upright position
B recurrent episodes of stridor are likely
C presentation typically occurs in adolescence
D recurrent pneumonia is a recognised complication
E dysphagia progressing over several months is typical

26
Typical features of sideropenic dysphagia include
A glossitis
B hyperchlorhydria
C splenomegaly
D hysterical personality
E mid-oesophageal web

27
Typical features of oesophageal achalasia include
A recurrent pneumonia
B spasm of the lower oesophageal sphincter with muscular hypertrophy
C heartburn and acid reflux
D predisposition to oesophageal carcinoma
E symptomatic response to pneumatic balloon dilatation

28
Paraoesophageal hiatus hernia
A is commoner than oeseophagogastric hiatus hernia
B occurs more often in elderly males than females
C typically presents with iron deficiency anaemia
D often causes incompetence of the lower oesophageal sphincter
E usually progresses to produce an oesophageal stricture

29
Oesophagogastric hiatus hernia
A occurs more frequently in elderly women than men
B usually presents with slowly progressive dysphagia
C invariably results in peptic oesophagitis
D associated with odynophagia suggests oesophageal carcinoma
E is best treated surgically when oesophagitis is severe

Answers
22 A C
23 B C E
24 A B D
25 B D

26 A C
27 A D E
28 none
29 A

30
In diffuse oesophageal spasm
A Auerbach's plexus is normal
B most patients are over the age of 60 years at presentation
C strong uncoordinated contractions occur unrelated to swallowing
D dysphagia is most often due to an associated oesophagitis
E cimetidine therapy typically reduces the frequency of chest pain

31
Oesophageal carcinoma in the UK
A is more common in men than women
B is most often due to adenocarcinoma
C typically produces dysphagia with a poorly localised level
D predominantly affects the upper third of the oesophagus
E is associated with alcohol and tobacco consumption

32
Typical features of oesophageal carcinoma at presentation include
A acid reflux and odynophagia
B painless obstruction to the passage of a food bolus
C weight loss attributable to metastatic disease
D metastatic spread in over 75%
E overall survival rates at 5 years of approximately 33%

33
Peptic ulcer disease in the UK
A affects 10% of the adult population and is increasing in incidence
B involves the stomach more often than the duodenum in females
C is commoner in Scotland than Southern England
D more often remits than relapses during pregnancy
E involving the duodenum is associated with blood group A

34
The following factors are known to be significantly associated with chronic duodenal ulcer disease
A oral contraceptive therapy
B duodenogastric reflux
C pernicious anaemia
D Helicobacter pyloris infection
E tobacco consumption

35
The following factors are known to the significantly associated with benign gastric ulcer disease
A duodenogastric reflux
B tobacco consumption
C gastric acid hypersecretion
D pernicious anaemia
E anti-inflammatory drug therapy

36
The following statements about peptic ulcer disease are true
A freedom from symptoms invariably indicates ulcer healing
B ulcer healing is delayed by tobacco consumption
C ulcer healing is promoted by the use of a bland diet
D localised epigastric pain with tenderness typifies an active ulcer
E relapse after cimetidine therapy usually indicates malignancy

37
In the treatment of chronic peptic ulceration
A sodium bicarbonate is the most efficacious of all antacids
B aluminium containing antacids produce diarrhoea
C magnesium containing antacids produce constipation
D bismuth compounds should not be used for maintenance therapy
E oesophagitis heals less readily than duodenitis

Answers
30 A B C
31 A E
32 B D
33 C D

34 D E
35 A B E
36 B D
37 D E

38
The agents listed below promote the healing of peptic ulcers by the following actions on gastric parietal cell function
A cimetidine — H$_2$ histamine receptor antagonist
B misoprostol — PGE$_2$ receptor agonist inhibits histamine effect
C omeprazole — hydrogen/potassium ion — ATP-ase inhibitor
D pirenzipine — acetyl choline receptor antagonist
E proglumide — gastrin receptor antagonist

39
Recognised indications for elective peptic ulcer surgery include
A recurrent ulcer despite previous peptic ulcer surgery
B chronic gastric ulcer persisting after 6 weeks medical therapy
C gastric outlet obstruction
D asymptomatic hour-glass deformity of the stomach
E persistently troublesome symptoms despite medical therapy

40
When elective peptic ulcer surgery is undertaken the following statements are true
A truncal vagotomy causes weight loss by inducing premature satiety
B truncal vagotomy delays gastric emptying and causes diarrhoea
C highly selective vagotomy usually denervates the small bowel
D vagotomy typically reduces gastric acid secretion by over 90%
E partial gastrectomy reduces the subsequent risk of gastric carcinoma

41
Gastroduodenal haemorrhage in the UK
A is more often due to chronic gastric ulcer than oesophageal varices
B has a 10% mortality when due to chronic peptic ulceration
C is a recognised complication of severe head injury
D is best investigated by endoscopy within 24 hours of admission
E is significantly associated with anti-inflammatory drug therapy

42
Typical features of major acute gastroduodenal haemorrhage include
A severe abdominal pain
B angor animi and restlessness
C syncope preceding other evidence of bleeding
D elevated blood urea and creatinine concentrations
E peripheral blood microcytosis

43
When acute gastroduodenal haemorrhage is suspected
A a pulse rate of 120/minute is most likely to be due to anxiety
B hypotension without a tachycardia suggests an alternative diagnosis
C the absence of anaemia suggests the volume of blood loss is modest
D naso-gastric aspiration provides an accurate estimate of blood loss
E endoscopy is best deferred pending blood volume replacement

---

Answers
38 A B C D E
39 C E
40 A B

41 A B C D E
42 B C
43 E

44
In resuscitating a patient with major gastroduodenal bleeding
A sedation is best avoided if the patient is hypotensive
B whole blood is preferable to packed red blood cells
C volume replacement with colloids is preferable to crystalloids
D monitoring the central venous pressure is unnecessary
E surgical intervention should be deferred in younger patients

45
Acute perforation of a peptic ulcer is typically associated with
A acute rather than chronic ulcers
B duodenal more often than gastric ulcers
C abdominal pain unrelated to the extent of peritoneal soiling
D the absence of nausea and vomiting
E symptomatic improvement several hours following onset

46
Characteristic features of gastric outlet obstruction include
A metabolic acidosis
B bile vomiting
C urinary pH < 5
D symptomatic relief after vomiting
E absent gastric peristalsis

47
In the treatment of gastric outlet obstruction
A surgical intervention is inevitably required
B intravenous fluids should include ammonium chloride solutions
C potassium replacement is best assessed by the urinary electrolytes
D gastric aspiration should always be undertaken prior to surgery
E parenteral vitamin therapy is usually unnecessary

48
Typical features of a gastrinoma (Z–E syndrome) include
A a small gastric tumour
B hepatic metastases at presentation
C parathyroid adenomas
D constipation
E absent response in acid secretion to pentagastrin stimulation

49
Recognised complications of peptic ulcer surgery include
A jejunal ulcer
B constipation
C biliary gastritis
D osteomalacia
E ulcerative colitis

50
Following gastric surgery for peptic ulcer disease
A osteoporosis develops within 5 years
B post-prandial discomfort is common
C anaemia does not occur after vagotomy alone
D iron deficiency is commoner than folate deficiency
E diarrhoea usually responds to tetracycline therapy

51
In the typical early post-cibal or dumping syndrome
A symptoms develop 1–2 hours after meals
B gastric emptying of liquids is delayed
C weakness, palpitation and sweating are due to hypoglycaemia
D small, iso-osmolar meals produce symptomatic improvement
E peripheral vasoconstriction is often marked

Answers
44 B C
45 B E
46 C D
47 D

48 B C E
49 A C D
50 B D
51 D

52
Acute gastritis is typically associated with
A Helicobacter pyloris infection
B pathognomonic appearances on barium radiology
C alcohol abuse
D elemental iron poisoning
E significant bleeding in renal failure

53
Chronic gastritis is typically associated with
A significant dyspepsia
B pernicious anaemia
C specific histopathology
D post-gastric surgery
E gastric carcinoma

54
Carcinoma of the stomach
A is commoner in the Western than the Eastern hemisphere
B is 100 times more common in patients with pernicious anaemia
C is associated with blood group O
D causes diarrhoea associated with rapid gastric emptying
E is a recognised complication following partial gastrectomy

55
Typical features of gastric carcinoma in the UK include
A progression to involve the duodenum
B origin within a chronic peptic ulcer
C overall 5 year survival rate of 25%
D folate deficiency anaemia
E supraclavicular lymphadenopathy

56
Recognised features of gastric carcinoma include
A presentation with ascites or an ovarian tumour
B peripheral blood tumour markers
C more favourable prognosis when arising in the gastric fundus
D acanthosis nigricans
E linitis plastica more obvious radiologically than endoscopically

57
The following statements about pancreatic function are true
A the islets of Langerhans comprise 10% of pancreatic cell mass
B 2–3 L of pancreatic exocrine fluid enters the duodenum daily
C secretin stimulates pancreatic trypsin secretion
D pancreatic polypeptide decreases pancreatic and biliary secretion
E pancreatic secretion in response to a protein meal is impaired in small bowel disease and following partial gastrectomy

58
In the investigation of chronic pancreatic disease
A glucose tolerance is typically normal in pancreatic carcinoma
B duodenal ileus is a characteristic feature of chronic pancreatitis
C stool microscopy is more helpful in adults than children
D ERCP can reliably distinguish carcinoma from chronic pancreatitis
E pancreatic calcification suggests that chronic pancreatitis is the result of alcohol abuse rather than biliary tract disease

---

Answers
52 A C D E
53 B C D E
54 D E
55 E

56 A D E
57 D E
58 E

59
Recognised causes of acute pancreatitis include
A mumps and Coxsackie B viral infections
B hypothermia and hyperlipidaemia
C gallstones in the common bile duct
D azathioprine therapy
E alcohol abuse

60
Typical features of acute pancreatitis include
A peripheral circulatory failure
B persistent diarrhoea
C pain radiating to the back
D pain relieved by vomiting
E obstructive jaundice

61
The following are characteristic of acute pancreatitis
A abdominal guarding develops soon after the onset of pain
B normal serum amylase concentration in the first 4 hours after onset
C persistent serum hyperamylaseaemia suggests a developing pseudocyst
D hypercalcaemia develops 5–7 days after onset
E hyperactive loud bowel sounds

62
In the management of acute pancreatitis
A early laparotomy is advisable to exclude alternative diagnoses
B opiates should be avoided because of spasm of the sphincter of Oddi
C intravenous fluids are unnecessary in the absence of a tachycardia
D the PaO_2 and central venous pressure should be monitored
E nasogastric aspiration is required since an ileus is inevitable

63
Recognised causes of chronic pancreatitis include
A hyperlipidaemia
B hypercalcaemia
C alcohol abuse
D pancreas divisum
E haemosiderosis

64
Typical features of chronic pancreatitis include
A back pain persisting for days or weeks
B decreased vitamin B_{12} absorption
C increased sodium concentration in the sweat
D abdominal pain occurring 12–24 hours after alcohol intake
E pancreatic calcification on plain abdominal X-rays

65
In the treatment of chronic pancreatitis
A diabetes mellitus responds well to sulphonylurea therapy
B surgery is contraindicated if the ampulla is stenosed
C opiate analgesics should be avoided given the risk of dependency
D cimetidine therapy impairs the efficacy of oral pancreatic enzymes
E fat-soluble vitamins should be given parenterally

66
Pancreatic pseudocysts are typically associated with
A an onset within 2 weeks of the onset of acute pancreatitis
B extension into the lesser sac of the peritoneal cavity
C peripheral blood leucocytosis and high serum amylase activity
D the development of stenosis of pancreatic ducts
E the disappearance of abdominal pain and vomiting

Answers
59 A B C D E
60 A C E
61 C
62 D E

63 A B C D
64 A B D E
65 none
66 A B C D

67
Cystic fibrosis of the pancreas
A is an autosomal dominant disorder
B is established by sweat sodium concentrations > 80 mmol/L
C produces neonatal small bowel obstruction
D is associated with a dysfunction of all mucus secreting glands
E produces cor pulmonale due to chronic bronchitis

68
Pancreatic carcinoma in the UK
A is decreasing in incidence
B is more common in males than females
C is associated with tobacco and alcohol consumption
D is associated with an overall 5 year survival rate of 20%
E is associated with metastatic spread in 33% at presentation

69
The typical features of pancreatic carcinoma include
A adenocarcinomatous histology
B origin in the body of the pancreas in 60% of cases
C abdominal pain when arising in the ampulla of Vater
D back pain and weight loss indicate a poor prognosis
E gallbladder enlargement when associated with gallstones

70
The following statements about small bowel absorption are true
A fat is chiefly absorbed in the terminal ileum
B fructose is absorbed by simple diffusion
C breath hydrogen concentration reflects small bowel lactase activity
D stool/serum alpha$_1$ antitypsin ratios assess protein absorption
E the absorption of bile acids reflects ileal function

71
The following statements about small bowel malabsorption are true
A gastro-enterostomy impairs intraluminal digestive processes
B bacterial small bowel colonisation reduces bile acid deconjugation
C 10 G of stool nitrogen per day indicates protein malabsorption
D cholestyramine is useful in the control of steatorrhoea
E impaired transport of nutrients from enterocytes in tropical sprue

72
In severe small bowel malabsorption the following investigations are often abnormal
A small bowel barium follow through radiology
B Lundh pancreatic stimulation test
C xylose absorption test
D bile acid and vitamin B$_{12}$ absorption tests
E activities of disaccharidases in small bowel mucosal biopsy

73
Recognised causes of small bowel malabsorption include
A hypothyroidism
B partial gastrectomy
C giardiasis
D Crohn's disease
E Meckl's diverticulum

74
In gluten enteropathy (Coeliac disease)
A the typical onset is in adolescence
B there is a predisposition to Hodgkin's lymphoma
C the toxic agent is the polypeptide alpha-gliadin
D gluten-free diets improve absorption but not the villous atrophy
E vitamin B$_{12}$ deficiency is usually responsible for anaemia

---

Answers
67 B C D
68 B C
69 A D
70 C E

.**71** A C
72 A B C D E
73 B C D
74 C

75
Tropical sprue is
A caused by altered sensitivity to rice
B associated with small bowel colonisation by Staphylococcus
C best treated with a lactose-rich gluten-free diet
D associated with the development of hypermagnesaemia
E likely to respond to oral tetracycline therapy

76
Typical clinical features of tropical sprue include
A generalised hyperpigmentation
B weight loss and abdominal distension
C cheilosis and stomatitis
D polyuria and nocturia
E folate and B_{12} vitamin deficiencies

77
Characteristic features of Crohn's disease include
A familial association with ulcerative colitis
B onset after the age of 50 years
C disease confined to the ileum and colon
D predisposition to renal and biliary calculi
E giant cell granulomata indistinguishable from TB

78
The typical clinical features of Crohn's disease include
A association with tobacco consumption
B diarrhoea is more severe than in ulcerative colitis
C presentation with sub-acute intestinal obstruction
D segmental involvement of the colon and rectum
E inflammation confined to the mucosa on histology

79
Recognised complications of Crohn's disease include
A pernicious anaemia
B erythema nodosum
C enteropathic arthritis
D aphthous mouth ulcers
E small bowel lymphoma

80
In the treatment of ileo-caecal Crohn's disease
A surgical bypass is preferable to localised resection
B antibiotic therapy should be avoided if at all possible
C corticosteroid therapy is contraindicated in the acute phase
D cholestyramine reduces the diarrhoea but increases steatorrhoea
E sulphasalazine reduces the risk of small bowel obstructon

81
Intestinal obstruction
A of mechanical type is a complication of inguinal hernia
B of paralytic type is a feature of peripheral circulatory failure
C from peritonitis is typically mechanical in type
D associated with strangulation is invariably mechanical in type
E of paralytic type eventually progresses to a mechanical type

82
In patients with intestinal obstruction
A vomiting is an invariable feature
B the rectum is usually collapsed and empty
C hyperactive loud bowel sounds suggest mechanical obstruction
D absent bowel sounds suggest a paralytic type of obstruction
E abdominal tenderness suggests strangulation or peritonitis

Answers
75 E
76 A B C D E
77 A D
78 A C D

79 B C D
80 D
81 A B
82 C D E

83
Acute peritonitis
A complicating appendicitis is typically caused by Esch. coli
B carries an overall mortality rate < 1% in the UK
C due to tuberculosis is usually blood-borne of pulmonary origin
D is invariably due to infection
E causes increasing abdominal rigidity as paralytic ileus develops

84
The following statements about intra-abdominal abscess are true
A pelvic abscess typically presents with urinary retention
B constipation is a typically early feature of pelvic abscess
C lower posterior chest tenderness suggests subphrenic abscess
D abscesses are best localised by abdominal ultrasonography
E antibiotic therapy alone should resolve a subphrenic abscess

85
Acute appendicitis
A typically commences with right iliac fossa pain
B is often associated with luminal obstruction of the appendix
C produces urinary symptoms simulating acute pyelonephritis
D typically produces constipation and persistent vomiting
E is usually associated with a temperature > 39 degrees C

86
In the diagnosis and treatment of acute appendicitis
A non-specific mesenteric adenitis often progresses to appendicitis
B recurrent abdominal pain suggests chronic appendicitis is likely
C rigors soon after the onset of pain make the diagnosis unlikely
D surgery should be avoided if the patient is pregnant
E immediate surgery is mandatory if an appendix mass is palpable

87
Characteristic features of ulcerative colitis include
A invariable involvement of the rectal mucosa
B segmental involvement of the colon and rectum
C pseudo-polyposis following healing of mucosal damage
D inflammation extending from the mucosa to the serosa
E entero-cutaneous and entero-enteric fistulae

88
Ulcerative colitis differs from Crohn's colitis in that
A the disease can occur at any age
B tobacco consumption is not associated with ulcerative colitis
C toxic dilatation only occurs in ulcerative colitis
D aphthous stomatitis is less common than in Crohn's disease
E colonic strictures do not occur in ulcerative colitis

89
Recognised complications of ulcerative colitis include
A pyoderma gangrenosum
B pericholangitis
C aphthous mouth ulcers
D colonic carcinoma
E enteropathic arthritis

Answers
83 A
84 C D
85 B C

86 C
87 A C
88 B D
89 A B C D E

90
In the treatment of severe acute ulcerative colitis
A antibiotic therapy is mandatory if the patient is febrile
B codeine phosphate increases the risk of toxic dilatation
C systemic corticosteroids induce a remission in the majority
D hypoproteinaemia indicates the need for albumin infusion
E failure of medical therapy indicates the need for surgery

91
In the maintenance treatment of ulcerative colitis
A corticosteroid therapy should be given orally
B sulphasalazine therapy reduces the risk of colonic carcinoma
C azathioprine will reduce corticosteroid maintenance therapy
D the onset of urticaria suggests an allergy to sulphasalazine
E unlike sulphasalazine, mesalazine produces headache and diarrhoea

92
Typical features of colonic diverticulosis in the UK include
A predominantly affects the right hemicolon
B predisposition to the development of colonic carcinoma
C better diagnosed by colonoscopy than by barium enema radiology
D reduction in the number of diverticula with a high fibre diet
E the absence of symptoms in the absence of complications

93
Typical features of colonic diverticulitis include
A severe rectal bleeding
B chronic iron deficiency anaemia
C septicaemia and paralytic ileus
D right iliac fossa pain
E vesico-colic fistula

94
The following statements about colonic polyps are true
A 75% of polyps occur in the right hemicolon
B the typical histology is that of tubular adenoma
C polyps > 2 cm in diameter are usually malignant
D intussusception is a recognised complication
E presentation with constipation is typical

95
Multiple polyposis
A is inherited as an autosomal recessive trait
B is usually clinically apparent before the age of 10 years
C left untreated, progresses to carcinoma before the age of 40 years
D is associated with gastric and small bowel polyps
E under the age of 20 is best treated with azathioprine

96
The following statements about colonic carcinoma are true
A it is the commonest of all gastrointestinal carcinomas
B the majority of carcinomas arise in the right hemicolon
C after resection, there is a recognised risk of a second carcinoma
D Duke's A classifies tumour extending to the serosa only
E only a minority of rectal tumours are palpable per rectum

Answers
90 B C E
91 C D
92 E

93 A C E
94 B C D
95 C D
96 A C

97
In colonic carcinoma
A of the caecum, presentation with iron deficiency anaemia is typical
B obstruction is typically an early event in carcinoma of the sigmoid
C metastatic spread is to the lungs rather than the liver
D concomitant multiple tumours are present in 20% of patients
E rising serum CEA levels post-resection suggest recurrent tumour

98
In Hirschsprung's diseases of the colon
A there is a female preponderance
B presentation typically occurs between the ages 3–5 years
C there is a segmental absence of the myenteric nerve plexus
D the rectum is typically loaded on digital examination
E the surgical treatment of choice is a defunctioning colostomy

99
The typical features of acute small bowel ischaemia include
A occlusion of the inferior mesenteric artery
B the recent onset of atrial fibrillation
C the sudden onset of abdominal pain, vomiting and diarrhoea
D peripheral circulatory failure and signs of peritonitis
E gaseous distension of the small bowel on plain abdominal X-rays

100
The typical features of acute ischaemic colitis include
A rigors, abdominal pain and constipation
B occlusion of the superior mesenteric artery
C profuse bloody diarrhoea and abdominal tenderness
D mucosal oedema with 'thumb-printing' on barium enema radiology
E resolution with the later development of a colonic stricture

101
The following statements about functional bowel disorders are true
A the typical symptoms affect 20% of apparently healthy adults
B only 25% of those affected seek medical advice
C they account for 50% of gastrointestinal outpatient referrals
D organic diagnoses are subsequently apparent in 25% of patients
E food intolerance is the likeliest explanation in most patients

102
The typical features of functional dyspepsia include
A nausea and epigastric distension
B abdominal pain and constipation
C tiredness and sleep disturbance
D vomiting and weight loss
E acid reflux and odynophagia

103
The typical features of the irritable bowel syndrome include
A nocturnal diarrhoea and weight loss
B onset after the age of 40 years
C history of abdominal pain in childhood
D right iliac fossa pain and urinary frequency
E abdominal distension, flatulence and pelletly stools

Answers
97 A B E
98 C
99 B C D

100 C D E
101 A B C
102 A B C
103 C D E

104
The management of functional bowel disorders should include
A antispasmodic and laxative drugs
B extensive investigations of aged < 30 years
C explanation and reassurance after a full examination
D evaluation of social and emotional factors
E referral for psychiatric assessment and therapy

Answers
104 C D

Diseases of the liver and biliary system

1
On examination of the liver
A the normal upper border lies at the 8th
   rib anteriorly
B percussion is useful in revealing a small
   liver
C the normal lower border extends below
   the xiphisternum
D a venous hum audible below the
   xiphisternum suggests a hepatoma
E arterial bruits invariably indicate the
   presence of tumour deposits

2
In the normal liver
A the space of Disse separates the
   hepatocytes from sinusoidal cells
B the hepatic artery supplies 50% of the
   total hepatic oxygen supply
C the portal vein supplies 65% of the total
   hepatic blood flow
D the left hepatic lobe contains the
   quadrate and caudate lobes
E the macrophages (Kupffer cells)
   comprise 2% of the hepatic cell mass

3
In hepatic protein metabolism
A alpha$_1$-foetoprotein is normally
   synthesised in the liver after birth
B alpha$_1$-antitrysin is metabolised in the
   gut after hepatic synthesis
C factor IX is the only clotting factor not
   synthesised in the liver
D most of the complement system
   components are hepatically synthesised
E urea synthesis from aminoacids occurs
   in both the liver and kidneys

4
In hepatic lipid metabolism
A serum lipid concentrations decrease in
   biliary obstruction
B most of the total body cholesterol is
   synthesised in the liver
C chylomicrons are synthesised exclusively
   in the liver
D serum lipoprotein lipase removes
   triglycerides from chylomicrons
E hepatic synthesis of lipoproteins
   increases in liver failure

5
In hepatic carbohydrate metabolism
A hepatic glycogen reserves are exhausted
   within 24 hours of fasting
B insulin stimulates the hepatic uptake of
   glucose absorbed after meals
C insulin suppresses hepatic lipolysis and
   glycogenolysis
D hepatic gluconeogenesis utilises
   pyruvate, glycerol and alanine
E most of the endogenous glucose
   production occurs in the muscles

6
Bilirubin
A is derived exclusively from the
   breakdown of haemoglobin
B in the unconjugated form is bound in the
   plasma to beta-globulin
C is conjugated in the microsomes of the
   hepatocytes
D diglucuronide is water-soluble and
   reabsorbed in the small bowel
E is normally excreted as stercobilinogen
   in the faeces and as the colourless
   urobilinogen in the urine

Answers
 1 B C
 2 A B C
 3 C D

 4 B D
 5 A B C D E
 6 C E

7
The concentration of conjugated bilirubin
A in the serum in haemolytic anaemia is typically increased

B in the urine of healthy subjects is typically undetectable

C normally constitutes most of the total serum bilirubin

D in the serum in Gilbert's syndrome is typically increased

E in the urine in viral hepatitis parallels that of urobilinogen

8
The following statements about bile acid metabolism are true
A 95% of bile acids excreted are reabsorbed in the terminal ileum

B primary bile acids recirculate through the gut 10 times per day

C faecal bile acids principally comprise secondary bile acids

D primary bile acids in the colon typically produce diarrhoea

E cholic and chenodeoxycholic acid are metabolised by colonic flora to deoxycholic and lithocholic acid respectively

9
The serum alanine aminotransferase (ALT) concentration
A is derived from a microsomal enzyme specific to hepatocytes

B is typically more than 5 times normal in alcoholic hepatitis

C is usually normal in both obstructive and haemolytic jaundice

D rises in parallel with the serum bilirubin in viral hepatitis

E like that of serum gamma-glutamyl transferase, typically increases in response to the intake of enzyme-inducing drugs

10
The serum alkaline phosphatase concentration
A is derived from the liver, bone, small bowel and placenta

B usually increases to more than 3 times normal in viral hepatitis

C derives mainly from hepatic sinusoidal and canalicular membranes

D is of particular prognostic value in chronic liver disease

E increases more in extrahepatic than intrahepatic cholestasis

11
When monitoring serum liver function values in liver disease
A the serum albumin falls rapidly in acute fulminant liver failure

B persistent hypergammaglobulinaemia indicates hepatocyte necrosis

C an increased IgA concentration is typical of alcoholic hepatitis

D the prothrombin time increases rapidly in severe acute hepatitis

E an increased IgG concentration suggests primary biliary cirrhosis

12
In the investigation of suspected liver disease
A ultrasonography will reliably distinguish solid from cystic masses

B radioisotope scanning will reliably exclude liver disease

C the anterior liver surface is not usually visible at laparoscopy

D the mortality rate of percutaneous liver biopsy is about 1%

E ascitic fluid protein concentrations > 30 G/L are compatible with the diagnoses of tuberculosis, carcinomatosis and hepatic vein thrombosis

---

Answers
  7 B
  8 ABCDE
  9 none

10 A C
11 C D
12 A E

13
The following statements about liver disease are true
A alcohol is a recognised cause of intrahepatic cholestasis
B night sweats are a recognised feature of hepatic metastases
C osteomalacia is a recognised feature of chronic obstructive jaundice
D jaundice and a palpable gallbladder suggest common bile duct stones
E serum unconjugated and conjugated bilirubin concentrations are both increased in acute viral hepatitis

14
In haemolytic jaundice in an adult
A the finding of serum bilirubin > 90 μmol/L is typical
B jaundice is often not evident unless the serum bilirubin > 50 μmol/L
C the urine is usually dark-brown due to the presence of urobilinogen
D the majority of patients have palpable splenomegaly
E the stools are characteristically pale

15
Characteristic features of Gilbert's syndrome include
A an autosomal recessive mode of inheritance
B decreased hepatic glucuronyl transferase activity
C unconjugated hyperbilirubinaemia < 100 μmol/L
D serum bilirubin concentration increased by fasting
E increased serum bile acid concentrations

16
Conjugated hyperbilirubinaemia is a typical finding in
A Dubin-Johnson syndrome
B Crigler-Najjar syndrome
C Rotor syndrome
D Gilbert's syndrome
E jaundice due to rifampicin

17
Acute hepatocellular jaundice is a recognised complication of exposure to the following agents
A isoniazid
B chlorpromazine
C Coxiella burnetii
D Helicobacter pylori
E Toxoplasma gondii

18
Acute cholestatic jaundice is a recognised adverse effect of
A chlorpropamide
B salicylates
C chlorpromazine
D methyl testosterone
E ethinyl oestradiol

19
The histopathological characteristics of viral hepatitis include
A polymorph leucocyte infiltration of the lobules
B sparing of the centrilobular areas
C collapse of the reticulin architecture
D hepatocyte necrosis with eosinophilic bodies
E fatty infiltration

20
The typical features of type A viral hepatitis (HAV) include
A RNA virus infection associated with seafood poisoning
B an incubation period of 3 months
C greater risk of fulminant liver failure in the young than the old
D headache, right hypochondrial pain and tenderness
E progression to chronic active hepatitis if cholestasis is prolonged

---

Answers
13 A B C E
14 B D
15 B C D
16 A C

17 A B C E
18 A C D E
19 C D
20 A D

21
The following statements about type A viral hepatitis are true
A persistent viraemia produces the post-hepatitis syndrome

B relapsing hepatitis usually indicates a poorer prognosis

C pancytopenia is a recognised complication following recovery

D drug-induced acute hepatitis produces identical liver histology

E travellers given immune serum globulin are protected for 3 months

22
The following features in a jaundiced patient would suggest extrahepatic cholestasis rather than viral hepatitis
A a palpable gallbladder and hepatomegaly

B right hypochondrial tenderness

C serum alkaline phosphatase concentration > 3 times normal

D marked pruritus and rigors

E peripheral blood polymorph leucocytosis

23
In the management of patients with acute viral hepatitis
A dietary protein and calorie intakes should be unrestricted

B alcohol should be avoided until the anorexia resolves

C bed rest is mandatory until the jaundice resolves

D immune serum globulin will shorten the duration of illness

E corticosteriod therapy should never be administered

24
The hepatitis B surface antigen (HBsAg) in the blood
A is detectable during the prodrome of acute type B hepatitis

B envelops a DNA viral particle transmissible in all body fluids

C persists in about 25% of adults following acute type B hepatitis

D is present in 50% of patients with hepatoma in the UK

E of apparently healthy subjects is found more commonly in Europe than in tropical countries

25
The typical features of type B viral hepatitis (HBV) include
A an incubation period of 1 month

B history of exposure to unsafe sex or drug abuse

C prodomal illness with polyarthralgia

D hepatitic illness more severe than with type A virus

E absence of progression to chronic active hepatitis

26
In non-A, non-B viral hepatitis (NANBV)
A the clinical features are similar to other viral hepatitides

B there are distinct parenteral and enteric forms (types C + E)

C the disease does not progress to chronic active hepatitis

D 1 month and 3 month incubation forms of the disease occur

E the viruses responsible produce 90% of all documented episodes of post-transfusion hepatitis in Europe and the USA

Answers
21 C D E
22 A C D E
23 A

24 A B
25 B D
26 A B D E

27
In delta or type D viral hepatitis (HDV)
A the infective agent is an RNA virus
B enteral and parenteral modes of transmission occur
C replication of the virus requires the presence of type B virus
D simultaneous infection with HBV often produces severe hepatitis
E pre-existing HBV carriage predisposes to the development of acute hepatitis or progression to chronic active hepatitis

28
The typical features of fulminant hepatic failure include
A onset within 8 weeks of the initial illness
B hepatosplenomegaly and ascites
C encephalopathy and foetor hepaticus
D nausea, vomiting and renal failure
E cerebral oedema without papilloedema

29
Typical liver function values in fulminant hepatic failure include
A hypoalbuminaemia
B hypoglycaemia
C prolonged prothrombin time
D serum alkaline phosphatase > 3 times normal
E peripheral blood lymphocytosis

30
The management of fulminant liver failure includes
A avoidance of dietary protein
B cimetidine therapy to prevent erosive gastritis
C fresh frozen plasma to correct coagulation disorders
D parenteral dextrose 10% to correct hypoglycaemia
E parenteral mannitol 20% to control cerebral oedema

31
The typical histopathology of persistent hepatitis includes
A lymphocytic infiltration limited to portal triads
B prominent hepatocytic changes with fatty infiltration
C destruction of the lobular architecture
D piecemeal necrosis of the liver parenchyma
E clinical correlation with chronic active hepatitis

32
The typical histopathology of aggressive hepatitis includes
A destruction of the lobular architecture
B porto-portal bridging with progression to cirrhosis
C inflammation extending from the portal tracts into the parenchyma
D spotty necrosis of small areas of the liver parenchyma
E clinical correlation with chronic persistent hepatitis

33
Typical clinical features of chronic persistent hepatitis include
A persistently severe nausea, anorexia and abdominal pain
B jaundice with hepatosplenomegaly
C normal serum bilirubin and alkaline phosphatase concentrations
D progression to chronic active hepatitis and cirrhosis
E persistent hepatitis histologically on liver biopsy

34
The clinical features of chronic active hepatitis include
A predominance of females aged 20–40
B acute onset simulating viral hepatitis in 25% of patients
C arthralgia, fever and amenorrhoea
D spider telangiectasia and hepatosplenomegaly
E Cushingoid facies, hirsutism and acne

Answers
27 A B C D E
28 A C D E
29 B C
30 A B C D E

31 A
32 A B C
33 C
34 A B C D E

35
Chronic active hepatitis associated with hepatitis B virus differs from that not associated with HBV infection in that
A it typically affects males over 30 years of age
B it often produces fulminant hepatic failure
C it is often characterised by florid physical signs
D it typically progresses slowly without exacerbations
E it is less likely to be complicated by hepatoma

36
Diseases associated with chronic active hepatitis include
A autoimmune haemolytic anaemia
B Hashimoto's thyroiditis
C type I diabetes mellitus
D Sjogren's syndrome
E rheumatoid arthritis

37
In suspected chronic active hepatitis the following serum tests 8 weeks after the onset of illness strongly support the diagnosis
A anti-nuclear and smooth muscle antibodies in high titres
B persistent alanine aminotranferase activity > 10 times normal
C hypoalbuminaemia with gammaglobulin > 2 times normal
D decreased caeruloplasmin concentration
E anti-mitochondrial antibodies in titres > 640

38
In the management of patients with chronic active hepatitis
A liver biopsy soon after the onset of the illness is vital
B remissions and relapses are characteristic
C associated with autoantibodies, 50% die within 5 years
D corticosteroid and azathioprine therapy is life-saving
E corticosteroids should be avoided in chronic HBV hepatitis

39
The typical features of adult hepatic cirrhosis include
A progressive hepatomegaly
B massive splenomegaly
C peripheral blood macrocytosis
D parotid gland enlargement
E gaseous abdominal distension

40
Hepatic cirrhosis in adults
A is cryptogenic in aetiology in 60% of patients
B is an early complication of severe acute type B viral hepatitis
C is a recognised complication of acute paracetamol poisoning
D due to alcohol is more likely in chronic than in episodic abuse
E is a recognised complication of kwashiorkor

41
Recognised features of hepatic cirrhosis include
A unilateral gynaecomastia
B libido which is decreased in males and increased in females
C hyperpigmentation due to cutaneous iron deposition
D Dupuytren's contracture due to the hypergammaglobulinaemia
E persistent mild fever and elevated blood sedimentation rate

---

Answers
35 A D
36 A B C D E
37 A B C

38 B D
39 C D E
40 B D
41 A E

42
In patients with hepatic cirrhosis
A central cyanosis results from pulmonary venoarterial shunting
B increasing jaundice suggests progressive liver failure
C the peripheral blood flow is typically reduced
D the glomerular filtration rate is decreased
E oesophageal varices indicate portal hypertension

43
In the investigation of hepatic cirrhosis
A normal liver function tests exclude the diagnosis
B the serum alkaline phosphatase is of useful prognostic value
C excess urobilinogen in the urine is a recognised feature
D abdominal distension invariably indicates ascites
E ascites is pathognomonic of portal hypertension

44
Hepatic encephalopathy due to progressive liver failure is suggested by the development of
A dysarthria and chorea
B day-night reversal in sleep pattern
C yawning and hiccoughing
D serum aminotransferase activity > 10 times normal
E epilepsy and disorientation

45
Hepatic encephalopathy in cirrhosis is typically precipitated by
A infection
B hypokalaemia
C abdominal surgery
D gastrointestinal bleeding
E magnesium trisilicate therapy

46
In the management of hepatic cirrhosis with ascites
A the dietary sodium intake should be restricted to 80 mmol/day
B paracentesis with salt-poor albumin improves the survival rate
C the daily calorie intake should be restricted to 1500 Calories
D diuretic therapy should achieve a weight loss of 2 Kg/day
E the dietary protein intake should be at least 80 G/day unless encephalopathy is suspected

47
The management of severe hepatic encephalopathy should include
A withdrawal of dietary protein intake
B lactulose to limit colonic ammonia absorption
C neomycin to reduce colonic bacterial flora
D diuretic therapy with potassium supplementation
E enteral or parenteral glucose 300 G/day

48
The hepatorenal syndrome in cirrhosis is characterised by
A acute renal tubular necrosis
B proteinuria and an abnormal urinary sediment
C urinary sodium concentration < 10 mmol/L
D urine/plasma osmolality ratio > 1.5
E renal tubular acidosis

Answers
42 A B D E
43 C
44 A B C E
45 A B C D

46 E
47 A B C E
48 C D

49
In the initial management of acute bleeding from oesophageal varices associated with hepatic cirrhosis
A there is a 50% mortality rate
B oesophageal sclerotherapy is not indicated
C intravenous vasopressin reduces portal venous pressure
D balloon tamponade is better deferred pending endoscopy
E oesophageal transection is contraindicated in hepatic failure

50
Contraindications to portal-systemic shunt surgery include
A age > 50 years
B splenomegaly without cirrhosis
C hypoalbuminaemia or overt jaundice
D varices which have never bled
E ascites or encephalopathy

51
In primary biliary cirrhosis
A middle-aged males are affected predominantly
B pruritus is invariably accompanied by jaundice
C osteomalacia and osteoporosis are often present
D lipid infiltration produces peripheral neuropathy
E serum smooth muscle antibodies are present in high titres

52
The typical features of primary biliary cirrhosis include
A xanthomata of the palmar creases and eyelids
B poor prognosis even in asymptomatic patients
C hepatomegaly preceding splenomegaly
D dilated bile ducts on ultrasonography
E improved survival rate with immunosuppressant therapy

53
The typical features of primary haemochromatosis include
A association with HLA A3
B male predominance
C hepatic cirrhosis and diabetes mellitus
D hypertrophic cardiomyopathy
E grey skin pigmentation due to ferritin deposition

54
The typical features of Wilson's disease include
A acute haemolytic anaemia
B acute hepatitis and chronic active hepatitis
C parkinsonian syndrome and hepatic cirrhosis
D osteomalacia and raised serum copper concentration
E renal tubular acidosis and Kayser-Fleischer rings

55
Recognised causes of portal hypertension include
A polycystic disease of the liver
B myeloproliferative disease
C hepatic schistosomiasis
D arsenic and vinyl chloride exposure
E hepatic vein obstruction (Budd-Chiari)

56
The typical features of the hepatic vein obstruction include
A predisposing disease in 75% of patients
B slow insidious onset of ascites
C abdominal pain and tender hepatomegaly
D hepatic venous obstruction on hepatic ultrasonography
E good response to anticoagulation

Answers
49 A C D
50 C D E
51 C D
52 A C

53 A B C
54 A B C E
55 A B C D E
56 C D

57
Diseases associated with hepatic vein obstruction include
A oral contraceptive therapy
B polycythaemia vera
C constrictive pericarditis
D hypernephroma
E aplastic anaemia

58
The typical features of congenital hepatic fibrosis include
A hypoalbuminaemic oedema
B presentation in adolescence with cysts
C renal failure due to polycystic renal disease
D portal hypertension and bleeding varices
E acute hepatitis in childhood

59
Primary hepatocellular carcinoma is associated with
A hepatic cirrhosis in 80% of patients in the UK
B ingestion of aflatoxin-contaminated food in the tropics
C haemochromatosis
D hepatitis A virus infection
E androgen and oestrogen ingestion

60
Typical complications of hepatocellular carcinoma include
A polycythaemia
B hyperglycaemia
C porphyria cutanea tarda
D hypocalcaemia
E Cushing's syndrome

61
The typical features of hepatocellular carcinoma include
A fever, weight loss and abdominal pain
B ascites and intra-abdominal bleeding
C venous hum over the liver
D serum alpha-foetoprotein in high titre
E surgically resectable disease in 50% of patients

62
Pyogenic liver abscesses are a recognised complication of
A ascending cholangitis
B Crohn's disease
C pancreatitis
D septicaemia
E peritonitis

63
The typical features of pyogenic liver abscess include
A obstructive jaundice and weight loss
B tender hepatomegaly without splenomegaly
C pleuritic pain and pleural effusion
D multiple abscesses especially in ascending cholangitis
E *Esch. coli., anaerobes* and streptococci present in pus

64
The following statements about biliary anatomy are true
A the right and left hepatic ducts join to form the common bile duct
B the normal common bile duct measures 10 mm in diameter
C the bile and pancreatic ducts usually join the duodenum separately
D the gallbladder is chiefly innervated by sympathetic nerves
E 1–2 litres of bile is secreted by the liver daily and concentrated 10-fold in the gall-bladder

Answers
57 A B C D E
58 C D
59 A B C E
60 A C

61 A B D
62 A B C D E
63 B C D E
64 E

65
Failure to opacify the gallbladder on an oral cholecystogram is a recognised occurrence in
A gastric outflow obstruction
B diarrhoea
C normal subjects
D jaundice
E malabsorption

66
Gallstones
A occur more frequently in black Africans and Indians than Caucasians
B are demonstrable in over 75% of UK patients > 60 years of age
C comprise cholesterol stones in 75% of gallstones in the UK
D are usually cholesterol stones in hepatic cirrhosis
E are usually the result of reduced hepatic bile acid secretion

67
Gallstones are a recognised complication of
A obesity
B oral contraceptive therapy
C chronic haemolytic anaemia
D terminal ileal disease
E drug therapy for hyperlipidaemia

68
The typical features of acute cholecystitis include
A absence of obstruction of the cystic duct
B sterile culture of bile 72 hours after onset
C invariable association with gallstones
D exacerbation of pain following morphine analgesics
E radio-opaque gallstones on plain X-ray

69
The typical clinical features of acute cholecystitis include
A jaundice, nausea and vomiting
B colicky abdominal pain in spasms lasting 2–5 minutes
C right hypochondrial tenderness worse on inspiration
D air in the biliary tree on plain X-ray
E peripheral blood leucocytosis

70
Recognised complications of gallstone disease include
A carcinoma of the gallbladder
B large bowel obstruction
C acute pancreatitis
D emphysematous cholecystitis
E mucocele and empyema of the gallbladder

71
The typical features of carcinoma of the gallbladder include
A preponderance of middle-aged males
B squamous tumour on histopathology
C the absence of gallstones
D gallbladder calcification on plain X-ray
E surgically resectable in the majority

72
The typical features of cholangiocarcinoma include
A association with hepatic cirrhosis
B abdominal pain and obstructive jaundice
C serum alpha-foetoprotein in high titre
D serum alkaline phosphatase > 3 times normal
E surgically resectable in the majority

Answers
65 A B C D E
66 E
67 A B C D E
68 none

69 C E
70 A C D E
71 D
72 B D

Diseases of the kidneys and genito-urinary system

1
The normal anatomy of the adult kidney includes
A innervation by the T10–T12 and L1 spinal roots
B 10–12 cm in length, 5–6 cm in width and 3–4 cm in thickness
C the left kidney lies below the level of the right kidney
D retroperitoneal position at the level of T12–L3 vertebra
E stationary in position throughout respiratory movements

2
In the normal renal blood supply at rest
A approximately 100,000 nephrons receive 1.2 L of blood per minute
B the afferent arterioles supply blood direct to the distal tubules
C the glomerular capillaries are supplied by the afferent arterioles
D the blood supply of the medulla arises from efferent arterioles
E the glomerular capillary filtration pressure is about 80 mmHg

3
Within the normal kidney
A 33% of the filtered water is reabsorbed in the proximal tubules
B ADH increases the water permeability of the distal tubules
C the glomerular filtrate contains about 200 mg protein per litre
D 33% of the filtered sodium is reabsorbed in the proximal tubules
E the juxtaglomerular apparatus comprises specialised cells of the efferent arterioles and proximal convoluted tubules

4
In the proximal convoluted tubules of the normal kidney
A 33% of filtered chloride is actively reabsorbed
B > 90% of filtered potassium is actively reabsorbed
C 66% of the filtered sodium is actively reabsorbed ·
D most of the filtered glucose is actively reabsorbed
E 33% of the filtered bicarbonate is passively reabsorbed

5
In the ascending limb of the loop of Henle in the medulla
A most of the remaining sodium is reabsorbed without water
B most of the remaining chloride is reabsorbed without water
C hydrogen ions are secreted in exchange for potassium ions
D ADH increases the reabsorption of water
E filtered bicarbonate is reabsorbed in exchange for chloride

6
In the distal convoluted tubules of the normal kidney
A sodium ions are reabsorbed with chloride ions
B sodium ions are reabsorbed in exchange for potassium or hydrogen
C the active secretion of potassium is controlled by aldosterone
D passive water loss is controlled by the effects of ADH
E ammonium is secreted once most of the bicarbonate is reabsorbed

Answers
1 ABD
2 CD
3 BC

4 BCD
5 AB
6 ABCDE

7
In the renal tubular control of normal acid-base balance
A 40–80 mmol of hydrogen ions are excreted in the urine per day
B ammonium secretion is increased by a vegetarian diet
C carbonic anhydrase in tubular cells controls hydrogen ion balance
D disodium hydrogen phosphate accepts 66% of excreted hydrogen ions
E bicarbonate reabsorption becomes incomplete once the plasma bicarbonate concentration exceeds 25 mmol/L

8
Congenital or acquired defects in renal tubular transport are a recognised cause of
A hypophosphataemia
B water intoxication
C hypoglycaemia
D hypokalaemia
E amino-aciduria

9
Renal tubular acidosis is associated with
A enhanced urinary acidification
B predisposition to hyperkalaemia
C Wilson's disease
D primary biliary cirrhosis
E chronic pyelonephritis

10
The kidney produces the following substances
A erythropoietin
B 25-hydroxy cholecalciferol
C prostaglandins PGE_2 and PGI_2
D angiotensin converting enzyme
E aldosterone

11
Oliguria is a typical feature of
A chronic pyelonephritis
B untreated cardiac failure
C prolonged hypokalaemia
D acute tubular necrosis
E Addison's disease

12
Polyuria is principally attributable to an osmotic diuresis in
A diabetes insipidus
B diabetes mellitus
C chronic renal failure
D thiazide diuretic therapy
E hyperparathyroidism

13
The urinary specific gravity
A is determined solely by the number of solute particles in solution
B is independent of the nature and quantity of dietary food intake
C principally reflects the urinary excretion of ammonium salts
D is increased by glycosuria to a greater degree than the osmolality
E achieved after an overnight fast should be > SG 1.021

14
The following statements about renal function are true
A free hydrogen ions are not normally excreted in the urine
B creatinine clearance is assessed using the formula $C = UV/P$
C urea clearance is a reliable estimate of glomerular filtration rate
D urinary pH < 5.4 is incompatible with a diagnosis of renal failure
E blood urea and creatinine concentrations usually rise in parallel

Answers
7 A C E
8 A D E
9 C D E
10 A C D

11 B D
12 B C D
13 D E
14 B

15
Urinary protein excretion
A comprising light chains is detectable by dipstix
B > 3 G/day is invariably due to glomerular disease
C in childhood is greater during the night than the day
D comprising myoglobin produces a positive dipstix test for blood
E comprises albumin alone in early diabetic nephropathy

16
Proteinuria > 3 G/day is a recognised feature of
A cardiac failure
B polycystic renal disease
C renal vein thrombosis
D minimal lesion glomerulonephritis
E chronic pyelonephritis

17
Microscopic haematuria is an expected finding in
A renal amyloidosis
B malignant hypertension
C membranous glomerulonephritis
D infective endocarditis
E renal infarction

18
Red-brown urinary discolouration in the absence of red blood cells on urine microscopy is a recognised feature of
A rifampicin therapy
B haemoglobinuria
C beeturia
D myoglobinuria
E acute porphyria

19
Urinary discolouration of the type described below results from the presence in the urine of the following chemicals
A orange urine — phenindione and phenolphthalein
B blue urine — tetracyclines and riboflavins
C grey-black urine — parenteral iron preparations
D brown urine — urobilinogen
E black urine — homogentesic acid

20
Typical features of the acute glomerulonephritis syndrome include
A bilateral renal angle pain and tenderness
B hypertension and periorbital facial oedema
C oliguria < 800 ml and haematuria
D highly selective proteinuria
E history of allergy with oedema of the lips

21
Typical features of the nephrotic syndrome include
A bilateral renal angle pain
B generalised oedema and pleural effusions
C hypoalbuminuria and proteinuria > 3 G/day
D hypertension and polyuria
E urinary sodium concentration > 20 mmol/L

22
Recognised presentations of glomerular disease include
A hypertension
B recurrent painless haematuria
C acute renal failure
D chronic renal failure
E asymptomatic proteinuria

Answers
15 B D E
16 C D
17 B D E
18 A B C D E

19 A C E
20 A B C
21 B C
22 A B C D E

23
Immune-complex glomerulonephritis is an expected feature of
A acute pyelonephritis
B acute hepatitis B virus infection
C systemic lupus erythematosus
D IgA nephropathy
E renal amyloidosis

24
Proliferative glomerulonephritis occurs in association with
A immune complex deposition on the glomerular basement membrane
B bacterial rather than viral infections
C infection with haemolytic streptococci more than any other bacteria
D haemoptysis in Goodpasture's syndrome
E a poorer prognosis in childhood than in adulthood

25
The typical histopathological features of proliferative glomerulonephritis include
A eosinophil glomerular infiltration
B mesangial cell proliferation
C epithelial crescent formation
D progressive glomerular fibrosis
E acute tubular necrosis

26
The following statements about acute proliferative glomerulonephritis are true
A a rise in diastolic blood pressure is found in < 25% of patients
B impaired urinary concentration is a typical early feature
C hypocomplementaemia is typical of post-streptococcal nephritis
D the cause of death in the acute phase is usually cardiac failure
E microscopic haematuria is invariable despite normal renal function

27
In the treatment of acute proliferative glomerulonephritis
A recovery is accelerated by dietary protein restriction
B corticosteroid therapy is contraindicated
C sodium restriction is usually unnecessary
D fluid restriction is mandatory when oedema is present
E hypertension usually responds to sodium restriction alone

28
IgA nephropathy is characterised by
A recurrent macroscopic haematuria in young adult males
B onset 14–21 days following respiratory tract infections
C nephrotic syndrome in 20% of patients
D progression to chronic renal failure occurs in 10% of patients
E diffuse mesangial proliferative glomerulonephritis on renal biopsy

29
Typical features of mesangiocapillary glomerulonephritis include
A presentation at the age 15–25 years
B hypertension and renal impairment at presentation
C good response to immunosuppressant therapy
D 10% progress to chronic renal failure
E an association with infective endocarditis

30
Typical causes of focal and segmental glomerulonephritis include
A Henoch-Schonlein purpura
B microscopic polyarteritis
C infective endocarditis
D Wegener's granulomatosis
E systemic lupus erythematosus

Answers
23 B C D
24 A C D
25 B C D
26 C D E

27 D E
28 A C D E
29 A B E
30 A B C D E

31
The characteristic features of crescentic glomerulonephritis are
A presentation with a nephrotic syndrome
B clinical course rapidly progressing to renal failure
C systemic lupus erythematosus is often present
D mesangial proliferation is usually absent on renal biopsy
E immunosuppressant therapy is usually successful in the majority

32
The typical features of Goodpasture's disease include
A circulating anti-glomerular basement membrane antibodies
B crescentic glomerulonephritis
C presentation in young adult males during the springtime
D haemoptysis and pulmonary infiltrates on chest X-ray
E acute renal failure unresponsive to immunosuppressant therapy

33
The characteristic features of membranous glomerulonephritis are
A absence of glomerular or mesangial cell proliferation histologically
B presentation with a nephrotic syndrome in middle aged males
C progression to hypertension and renal failure in 50% of patients
D association with HLA B8 and DRw3 confers a good prognosis
E treatment with immunosuppression is useful in the majority

34
Membranous glomerulonephritis is a recognised complication of
A renal amyloidosis
B bronchial carcinoma
C lymphoma
D malaria and hepatitis B infections
E polyarteritis nodosa

35
Characteristic features of minimal lesion glomerulonephritis are
A occurrence in adults after intercurrent infections
B mesangial cell proliferation on renal biopsy
C nephrotic syndrome with unselective proteinuria
D hypertension and microscopic haematuria
E renal impairment in association with HLA B12 and DRw7

36
In the treatment of minimal lesion glomerulonephritis
A therapy should be deferred pending renal biopsy in childhood
B diuretics should be avoided to minimise the risk of renal impairment
C following corticosteroid therapy, 30% relapse within 3 years
D immunosuppressant therapy is indicated for frequent relapses
E deterioration in renal function commonly develops in the long term

37
Renal involvement in systemic lupus erythematosus
A is clinically apparent in 40% at presentation
B is invariably apparent on renal biopsy in patients with SLE
C usually comprises diffuse proliferative glomerulonephritis
D has a poor prognosis in patients with membranous glomerulonephritis
E is typical of drug-induced SLE

Answers
31 B D
32 A B C D E
33 A B C
34 B C D

35 none
36 C D
37 A B C

38
Renal amyloidosis is characteristically associated with
A acute proliferative glomerulonephritis syndrome
B nephrogenic diabetes insipidus
C renal tubular acidosis
D progression to renal failure in 50% within 6 months
E myelomatosis

39
The typical features of lower urinary tract infections include
A rigors, loin pain and renal impairment
B suprapubic pain, dysuria and haematuria
C progression to acute pyelonephritis if untreated
D midstream urine culture producing *Esch. coli* > 100,000 /ml
E relief of dysuria with oral ammonium chloride therapy

40
The typical features of acute pyelonephritis include
A normal anatomy of the urinary tract
B vomiting, rigors and renal angle tenderness
C renal angle pain is invariably bilateral
D septicaemia and peripheral blood leucocytosis
E dysuria, haematuria and pyuria

41
Recognised complications of acute pyelonephritis include
A strangury
B septicaemia
C necrotising papillitis
D acute renal failure
E oedema of the loin

42
Conditions which predispose to acute pyelonephritis include
A vesico-ureteric reflux
B pregnancy
C diabetes mellitus
D analgesic abuse
E renal calculi

43
During the first trimester of pregnancy
A asymptomatic bacteriuria is present in 20% of patients
B ureteric atonia predisposes to the onset of acute pyelonephritis
C treatment of asymptomatic bacteriuria prevents symptom onset
D intravenous urography is mandatory given acute pyelonephritis
E cotrimoxazole is the treatment of choice in acute cystitis

44
The typical features of renal tuberculosis include
A presentation with bilateral loin pain
B renal medullary involvement precedes renal cortical involvement
C recurrent haematuria and sterile pyuria
D ascending infection from bladder tuberculosis
E concurrent corticosteroid and anti-TB therapy is contraindicated

45
The following statements about chronic pyelonephritis are true
A it is a recognised association of nephrocalcinosis
B it can be reliably distinguished from analgesic nephropathy
C the prognosis is worse in paraplegic and diabetic patients
D renal impairment usually only develops after the age of 50 years
E it is a recognised cause of chronic sodium depletion

Answers
38 B C D E
39 B D
40 B D E
41 A B C

42 A B C D E
43 B C
44 C
45 A C E

46
Chronic pyelonephritis in adults
A accounts for 80% of patients requiring chronic dialysis in the UK
B is usually attributable to vesico-ureteric reflux in childhood
C commonly presents with hypertension and chronic renal failure
D is usually associated with demonstrable ureteric reflux
E with hypertension should be treated with oral sodium chloride

47
Chronic renal failure is a recognised complication of
A congenital polycystic kidneys
B malignant hypertension
C proliferative glomerulonephritis
D juvenile chronic pyelonephritis
E schistosomiasis

48
Recognised complications of chronic renal failure include
A macrocytic anaemia
B peripheral neuropathy
C bone pain
D polyuria
E metabolic alkalosis

49
Typical biochemical features of chronic renal failure include
A impaired urinary concentration and dilution
B hypophosphataemia
C hypercalcaemia
D metabolic acidosis
E proteinuria > 3 G/L

50
Adverse prognostic features in chronic renal failure include
A papilloedema
B urinary granular casts
C enterocolitis
D renal osteodystrophy
E serum creatinine > 300 umol/L

51
The following statements about dialysis and transplantation are true
A peritoneal dialysis is preferable to haemodialysis in childhood
B the 5 year mortality rate for haemodialysis is approximately 5%
C peritoneal dialysis (CAPD) is contraindicated in diabetic patients
D renal graft survival is influenced more by ABO than HLA compatibility
E the 5 year renal graft survival is approximately 25%

52
The typical features of acute renal failure include
A oliguria < 800 ml/day is invariably present
B renal ischaemia is invariably associated with systemic hypotension
C urinary osmolality > 600 mosmol/Kg indicates acute tubular necrosis
D urinary sodium concentration < 20 mmol/L indicates irreversibility
E anaemia with a haemoglobin concentration < 80 G/L

53
Recognised causes of acute renal failure include
A septicaemia
B cardiac failure
C eclampsia
D acute tubulo-interstitial nephritis
E disseminated intravascular coagulation

Answers
46 B C
47 A B C D E
48 B C D
49 A D

50 A C D E
51 A D
52 none
53 A B C D E

54
The treatment of the oliguric phase of acute renal failure includes
A restriction of dietary protein to 40 G/day
B calcium resonium orally and/or rectally to reduce hyperkalaemia
C restriction of fluid intake to the total volume of daily losses
D tetracycline therapy if enterocolitis supervenes
E avoidance of dialysis if pulmonary oedema supervenes

55
Haemofiltration in the oliguric phase of acute renal failure is
A particularly useful when parenteral nutrition is required
B contraindicated in patients with cardiac failure
C preferable to peritoneal dialysis in young children
D usually undertaken on a 24-hour basis for 10–20 days
E more effective than peritoneal dialysis in restoring acid-base balance

56
During the diuretic phase of acute renal failure
A the blood urea concentration decreases rapidly
B increases in the dietary protein intake should be avoided
C sodium, potassium and bicarbonate supplementation is required
D fluid restriction should be maintained
E renal medullary dysfunction typically persists for 2–3 months

57
In post-renal acute renal failure
A unilateral obstruction suggests non-function of the other kidney
B anuria is less common than in acute tubular necrosis
C surgical intervention should be deferred until the blood urea falls
D antegrade pyelography and percutaneous nephrostomy are mandatory
E relief of the obstruction is usually followed by persistent oliguria

58
The typical features of acute tubulo-interstitial nephritis include
A skin rashes, arthralgia and bone marrow depression
B absence of a peripheral blood eosinophilia
C renal biopsy evidence of an eosinophilic interstitial nephritis
D renal impairment is invariable following drug withdrawal
E onset following antibiotic or anti-inflammatory drug therapy

59
Ureteric obstruction
A predisposes to stone formation
B is a recognised complication of cervical carcinoma
C unlike bladder-neck obstruction, seldom causes haematuria
D at the pelvi-ureteric junction in childhood is usually congenital
E is invariably painfree if the onset is gradual

60
Disorders predisposing to renal stone formation include
A urinary tract infection
B prolonged immobilisation
C hypoparathyroidism
D renal tubular acidosis
E Cushing's syndrome

Answers
54 B C
55 A D
56 C

57 A D
58 A C E
59 A B D
60 A B D E

61
Renal calculi in the UK
A predominantly occur in elderly women
B most often comprise calcium oxalate and calcium phosphate
C due to uric acid occur more often in alkaline than acid urine
D are typically asymptomatic until they migrate into the ureters
E associated with nephrocalcinosis is typical of sarcoidosis

62
Renal pain
A is typically localised to the iliac fossa
B caused by ureteric calculus is due to a rise in intra-renal pressure
C is characteristically absent in polycystic renal disease
D associated with rigors suggests acute pyelonephritis
E due to renal pelvic carcinoma usually indicates metastatic spread

63
In the treatment of renal calculi
A anuria indicates the need for urgent surgical intervention
B the urine should be alkalinised if the stone is radio-opaque
C bendrofluazide increases urinary calcium excretion
D allopurinol increases urinary urate excretion in gouty patients
E allopurinol decreases stone formation in idiopathic hypercalciuria

64
The clinical features of adult polycystic renal disease include
A an autosomal recessive mode of inheritance
B cystic disease of the liver and pancreas
C renal angle pain and haematuria
D unilateral renal enlargement
E aneurysms of the circle of Willis

65
Characteristic features of renal tubular acidosis (RTA) include
A normal anion gap
B hyperchloraemic acidosis
C inappropriately high urinary pH > 5.4
D decreased glomerular filtration rate
E normocytic normochromic anaemia

66
Recognised causes of proximal type II RTA include
A amyloidosis
B heavy metal poisoning
C renal transplant rejection
D hyperparathyroidism
E medullary sponge kidney

67
Recognised causes of distal type I RTA include
A lithium therapy
B hyperparathyroidism
C Sjogren's syndrome
D renal transplant rejection
E chronic pyelonephritis

68
Recognised causes of distal type IV RTA include
A Addison's disease
B spironolactone therapy
C isolated primary hypoaldosteronism
D hyporeninaemic hypoaldosteronism in diabetic nephropathy
E hyporeninaemic hypoaldosteronism in hypertensive nephrosclerosis

Answers
61 B D E
62 D
63 A E
64 B C E

65 A B C
66 A B C
67 A B C D E
68 A B C D E

69
The typical features of distal type I RTA include
A impaired renal tubular reabsorption of bicarbonate
B hyperchloraemic acidosis
C renal sodium wasting and hypokalaemia
D osteomalacia, hypophosphataemia and hypercalciuria
E autosomal recessive mode of inheritance in the familial form

70
The typical features of proximal type II RTA include
A impaired renal tubular secretion of hydrogen ions
B hyperchloraemic acidosis and hypokalaemia
C glycosuria, uricosuria and aminoaciduria
D hypocalcaemia and hypophosphataemia
E urinary pH which cannot be reduced to pH < 5.5

71
The typical features of distal type IV RTA include
A normal renal tubular secretion of hydrogen and potassium ions
B hyperchloraemic acidosis and hyperkalaemia
C decreased glomerular filtration rate
D increased anion gap and aminoaciduria
E good response to fludrocortisone therapy

72
The typical features of analgesic nephropathy include
A renal disease exclusively attributable to phenacetin
B acute papillary necrosis with recurrent renal colic
C tubular atrophy and fibrosis due to renal medullary ischaemia
D microscopic haematuria and sterile pyuria
E oliguria associated with urinary tract infections

73
Renal excretion of the following drugs is impaired in renal failure
A cimetidine
B tetracycline
C digoxin
D morphine
E co-trimoxazole

74
Recognised features of renal carcinoma include
A persistent fever
B bone metastases
C haematuria with renal colic
D polycythaemia
E serum alpha-foetoprotein in high titre

75
The following statements about the urinary bladder are true
A tabes dorsalis produces incontinence with painless over-distension
B prolapsed lumbar vertebral disc usually produces urinary urgency
C pneumaturia is most often the result of severe bladder sepsis
D urinary stress incontinence suggests cerebrovascular disease
E urinary retention is an expected complication of opiate therapy

76
Typical features of bladder carcinoma include
A squamous cell rather than transitional cell in origin
B presentation with urinary frequency and nocturia
C unresponsive to radiotherapy
D early metastatic spread to the liver and lungs
E association with exposure to dyes and tobacco consumption

Answers
69 B C D
70 B C D
71 B C
72 B C D

73 A C D E
74 A B C D
75 A E
76 E

77
Typical features of prostatic carcinoma include
A slowly progressive obstructive uropathy
B presentation with urinary frequency and nocturia
C preservation of the normal anatomy on digital rectal examination
D local spread along the lumbosacral nerve plexus
E osteoporotic rather than osteosclerotic bone metastases

78
The typical features of benign prostatic hypertrophy include
A peak incidence in the age group 40–60 years
B acute urinary retention and haematuria
C increased plasma testosterone concentration
D normal serum prostatic acid phosphatase concentration
E asymmetrical prostatic enlargement on rectal examination

79
During examination of the male genitalia
A nodular enlargement of the testis suggests tuberculosis
B hypospadias is a recognised finding in 5% of normal males
C mumps infection usually produces thickening of the epididymis
D the spermatic cord is typically lengthened in testicular torsion
E the finding of a hydrocele usually excludes testicular tumour

80
Characteristic features of testicular tumours include
A testicular pain in seminoma of the testis
B alpha-foetoprotein and chorionic gonadotrophin secretion in teratomas
C serum placental alkaline phosphatase present in 40% of seminomas
D peak incidence in males aged 40–60 years
E seminomas but not teratomas are both radio- and chemo-sensitive

---

Answers
77 A B D
78 B D

79 none
80 B C

Endocrine and metabolic diseases

1
The following hypothalamic releasing factors stimulate the pituitary gland to secrete the hormones listed below
A dopamine — prolactin
B somatostatin — growth hormone
C thyrotrophin releasing hormone (TRH) — TSH and prolactin
D gonadotrophin releasing hormone (GnRH) — LH and FSH independently
E corticotrophin releasing hormone (CRH) — beta-lipotrophin and ACTH

2
The following statements about pituitary tumours are true
A chromophobe adenomas typically produce hypopituitarism
B diabetes insipidus usually indicates supra-sellar extension
C Cushing's disease is usually caused by acidophilic macroadenomas
D acromegaly is most often associated with basophilic microadenomas
E tumour enlargement with expansion of the pituitary fossa usually presents with headaches and/or a bitemporal upper quadrantanopia

3
The typical features of acromegaly include
A thoracic kyphosis and myopathy
B hypertension and diabetes mellitus
C goitre and cardiomegaly
D growth hormone suppression during a glucose tolerance test
E hyperhydrosis

4
The typical features of pituitary-dependent Cushing's disease include
A enlargement of the pituitary fossa
B amenorrhoea and depression
C proximal myopathy and diabetes mellitus
D suppression of plasma cortisol following dexamethasone
E hypotension and hyperkalaemia

5
Recognised causes of hyperprolactinaemia include
A oestrogen therapy
B chlorpromazine and haloperidol therapy
C primary hypothyroidism
D hypoadrenalism
E Cushing's disease

6
In childhood growth hormone deficiency
A panhypopituitarism is a typical finding
B most patients have a craniopharyngioma
C a genetic deficiency of GH releasing factor is common
D delayed bone development is a characteristic feature
E treatment with human growth hormone produces precocious puberty

7
Recognised causes of short stature in childhood include
A Klinefelter's syndrome
B Turner's syndrome
C emotional deprivation
D Cushing's syndrome
E hyperthyroidism

Answers
1 C D E
2 A B E
3 A B C E

4 B C
5 A B C D E
6 C D
7 B C D

8
Recognised causes of hypopituitarism include
A post-partum haemorrhage
B Cushing's syndrome
C acromegaly
D autoimmune hypophysitis
E sarcoidosis

9
The clinical features of hypopituitarism include
A hypotension with hyperkalaemia
B a normal increment in plasma cortisol 30 minutes after i.v. ACTH
C loss of libido, menstruation and secondary sexual hair
D hypoglycaemia without the typical symptoms
E coma and water intoxication

10
The typical features of cranial diabetes insipidus include
A serum sodium concentration > 150 mmol/L with urine SG < 1.001
B increased polyuria following corticosteroid therapy for hypopituitarism
C onset following basal meningitis or hypothalamic trauma
D decreased renal responsiveness to ADH following carbamazepine therapy
E unlike psychogenic polydipsia, the response to ADH is normal

11
Recognised causes of nephrogenic diabetes insipidus include
A lithium therapy
B heavy metal poisoning
C congenital sex-linked recessive disorder
D chlorpropamide therapy
E hyperkalaemia and hypocalcaemia

12
Recognised causes of inappropriate ADH secretion include
A meningitis
B head injury
C lobar pneumonia
D small cell bronchial carcinoma
E phenothiazine and amitriptyline therapy

13
The following statements about thyroid hormones are true
A T3 and T4 are both stored in colloid vesicles as thyroglobulin
B T4 is metabolically more active than T3
C T3 and T4 are mainly bound to albumin in the serum
D 85% of the circulating T3 arises from extra-thyroidal T4
E reverse-T3 is a potent inhibitor of T4 conversion to T3

14
The finding of reduced serum total T3, total T4 and TSH concentrations is compatible with the following conditions
A hypopituitarism
B primary hypothyroidism
C nephrotic syndrome
D liver failure
E pregnancy

15
The following thyroid function tests invariably indicate significant disease of the thyroid gland
A decreased serum total T4 and TSH concentrations
B increased serum free T4 and decreased TSH concentrations
C decreased serum free T4 without a rise in TSH after i.v. TRH
D decreased serum total T4 and TSH with TSH receptor antibodies
E decreased serum free T4 and increased TSH concentrations

Answers
 8 A C D E
 9 C D E
10 B C E
11 A B C

12 A B C D E
13 A D E
14 A C D
15 B D E

16
The following statements about thyrotoxicosis are true
A type I is typically associated with serum TSH receptor antibodies
B in type II a solitary 'hot' nodule is typically present
C type III is associated with multinodular goitre in older patients
D in type I (Graves' disease) the thyroid gland is diffusely hyperactive
E there is an increased prevalence of HLA-DR3 in Graves' disease

17
The clinical features of thyrotoxicosis include
A atrial fibrillation with a collapsing pulse
B weight loss and oligomenorrhoea
C peripheral neuropathy
D proximal myopathy and exophthalmos
E decreased insulin requirements in type I diabetes mellitus

18
In the treatment of thyrotoxicosis
A propranolol should not be given in atrial fibrillation
B carbimazole blocks the secretion of T3 and T4 by the thyroid
C persistent suppression of the serum TSH is an indication for surgery
D serum TSH receptor antibodies usually persist despite carbimazole
E surgery is more likely to be necessary in young men than young women

19
Following ^{131}I radioiodine treatment for thyrotoxicosis
A transient hypothyroidism invariably produces an elevated serum TSH
B at least 50% of patients develop hypothyroidism within 7 years
C relapse is common in patients with a solitary 'hot' nodule
D 50% of the thyroidal isotope uptake is still present 8 days later
E 70% of patients require further ^{131}I

20
The following regimens would be appropriate in the management of a 30 year old woman with severe thyrotoxic Graves' disease
A carbimazole with ^{131}I radioiodine
B potassium perchlorate with carbimazole
C propranolol with carbimazole
D subtotal thyroidectomy following thyrotoxic control
E prednisolone with potassium iodide and propranolol

21
Complications of subtotal thyroidectomy for thyrotoxicosis include
A transient hypothyroidism
B recurrent laryngeal nerve palsy
C hypoparathyroidism
D recurrent thyrotoxicosis
E thyroid carcinoma

22
In Graves' ophthalmopathy
A both eyes are invariably affected
B the patient is invariably thyrotoxic
C serum eye muscle antibodies are pathognomonic
D in 90% of patients the condition resolves spontaneously
E hypothyroidism exacerbates the condition

23
The clinical features of primary hypothyroidism include
A carpal tunnel syndrome and proximal myopathy
B cold sensitivity and menorrhagia
C deafness and dizziness
D puffy eyelids and malar flush
E absent ankle tendon reflexes

Answers
16 A D E
17 A B D
18 E
19 B D

20 C D E
21 A B C D
22 D E
23 A B C D

24
Biochemical findings in primary hypothyroidism include
A low serum free T3 preceding an increase in serum TSH concentration
B increased serum prolactin concentration
C inappropriate ADH secretion
D increased serum alkaline phosphatase concentration
E increased serum cholesterol concentration

25
Clinical features of primary hypothyroidism in childhood include
A malabsorption with diarrhoea
B precocious puberty
C retardation of growth and sexual development
D epiphyseal dysgenesis on bone X-rays
E permanent mental retardation

26
Recognised causes of goitre include
A acromegaly
B lithium and amiodarone therapy
C Hashimoto's thyroiditis
D oral contraceptive therapy and pregnancy
E Pendred's syndrome (thyroidal dyshormonogenesis)

27
The following statements about goitre are true
A elevation of the ESR favours a diagnosis of thyroid carcinoma
B hypothyroidism favours a diagnosis of Hashimoto's thyroiditis
C deafness in childhood suggests a diagnosis of dyshormonogenesis
D episodic facial flushing and diarrhoea suggests hyperthyroidism
E serum thyroid antibodies favour a diagnosis of subacute thyroiditis

28
Typical features of de Quervain's subacute thyroiditis include
A large painless goitre
B giant cells on histopathology
C clinical signs of hyperthyroidism
D elevated ESR and serum thyroid antibodies
E goitre regression following thyroxine therapy

29
The development of a simple colloid goitre is associated with
A Coxsackie B viral infection
B dietary iodine deficiency
C excess dietary calcium intake
D Turner's syndrome
E dietary goitrogens

30
Thyroid carcinoma
A usually presents as a single 'hot' thyroid nodule
B of anaplastic type is usually cured by local radiotherapy
C of follicular type is best treated by ^{131}I radioiodine therapy alone
D of papillary type should be treated with total thyroidectomy
E of medullary type usually presents with episodic flushing and diarrhoea

31
The plasma ionised calcium concentration is typically increased in
A hypoalbuminaemia
B pyloric stenosis
C carcinomatosis
D hypoparathyroidism
E chronic sarcoidosis

Answers
24 B C E
25 B C D
26 A B C D E
27 B C

28 B E
29 B C E
30 D E
31 C E

32
Typical clinical features of primary hyperparathyroidism include
A recurrent acute pancreatitis and renal colic due to calculi
B hyperplasia of all the parathyroid glands on histology
C osteitis fibrosa on bone X-rays at presentation
D the complications of pseudo-gout and hypertension
E renal tubular acidosis and nephrogenic diabetes insipidus

33
Typical biochemical findings in primary hyperparathyroidism include
A increased serum calcium and phosphate concentrations
B decreased serum 1,25-dihydroxycholecalciferol concentration
C hypercalciuria and hyperphosphaturia
D increased serum alkaline phosphatase with bony involvement
E increased serum calcium and PTH concentrations

34
Recognised features of secondary hyperparathyroidism include
A calcification of the basal ganglia
B complication of chronic renal failure
C parathyroid enlargement is typically palpable
D development of parathyroid adenomas
E complication of gluten enteropathy

35
Recognised features in type I multiple endocrine neoplasia (MEN) include
A sex-linked recessive mode of inheritance
B hypercalcaemia, hypergastrinaemia and hyperprolactinaemia
C medullary thyroid carcinoma, phaeochromocytoma and parathyroid adenoma
D neurofibromata, phaeochromocytoma and medullary thyroid carcinoma
E insulinoma, pituitary adenoma and parathyroid adenoma

36
Recognised causes of hypercalcaemia include
A bone metastases secreting prostaglandins
B carcinomas secreting PTH-like peptides
C severe Addison's disease
D severe hypothyroidism
E immobilisation in Paget's disease

37
The clinical features of hypoparathyroidism include
A carpopedal and laryngeal spasm
B fungal infection of the finger nails
C abdominal pain and constipation
D peripheral paraesthesiae and psychosis
E cataracts and epilepsy

38
Recognised causes of hypoparathyroidism include
A autoimmune disease often also involving other endocrine glands
B Di George's syndrome with congential thymic aplasia
C subtotal thyroidectomy for thyrotoxicosis
D medullary carcinoma of the thyroid gland
E metastatic disease within the thyroid gland

Answers
32 A D E
33 C D E
34 B D E

35 B E
36 A B C E
37 A B D E
38 A B C

39
The typical features of pseudohypoparathyroidism include
A impaired coupling of adenyl cyclase with the renal PTH receptor
B decreased serum PTH and calcitonin concentrations
C decreased serum calcium and phosphate concentrations
D family history of short stature and growth retardation
E mental retardation and shortening of the metacarpals 4 and 5

40
Recognised causes of tetany due to hypocalcaemia include
A hyperventilation
B pyloric stenosis
C primary hyperaldosteronism
D acute pancreatitis
E gluten enteropathy

41
In the treatment of primary hypoparathyroidism
A intravenous calcium gluconate should be given if tetany develops
B intranasal PTH therapy should be given longterm
C calcitonin therapy prevents the onset of cataracts
D oral 1 alpha-hydroxycholecalciferol restores calcium homeostasis
E 5% carbon dioxide inhalation is required if tetany develops

42
The following statements about adrenal gland physiology are true
A ACTH normally controls the adrenal secretion of aldosterone
B ACTH increases adrenal androgen and cortisol secretion
C the plasma cortisol concentration normally peaks in the evening
D hyperglycaemia increases the rate of cortisol secretion
E cortisol enhances gluconeogenesis and lipogenesis from amino acids

43
A typical Cushingoid appearance is an expected finding in
A chronic alcohol abuse
B pituitary macrodenomas
C ACTH-secreting bronchial carcinoma
D adrenocortical adenoma
E fludrocortisone therapy

44
Oral cortiscosteroids are more likely than ACTH therapy to produce
A exacerbations of peptic ulcer disease
B growth retardation in childhood
C skin pigmentation
D acne vulgaris
E Cushingoid facies

45
The typical clinical features of Cushing's syndrome include
A generalised osteoporosis
B systemic hypotension
C hirsutism and amenorrhoea
D proximal myopathy
E hypoglycaemic episodes

Answers
39 A D E
40 D E
41 A D

42 B E
43 A D
44 B
45 A C D

46
Expected findings in patients with benign adrenal adenomas include
A preservation of the normal diurnal rhythm of cortisol secretion
B plasma cortisol < 170 nmol/L 10 hours after 2 mg dexamethasone orally
C increased free cortisol/creatinine ratios in early-morning urine
D increased plasma dehydroepiandrosterone concentrations
E increased plasma 17 alpha-hydroxyprogesterone concentrations

47
In primary hyperaldosteronism (Conn's syndrome)
A peripheral oedema is usually present
B proximal myopathy is due to hypokalaemia
C polyuria and polydipsia are characteristic
D diabetes mellitus is often present
E hypertension is associated with hypereninaemia

48
Recognised causes of primary adrenocortical insufficiency include
A haemochromatosis
B autoimmune adrenalitis
C amyloidosis
D sarcoidosis
E tuberculosis

49
Typical features of primary adrenocortical insufficiency include
A anorexia, weight loss and diarrhoea
B pigmentation of scars present before the onset of hypoadrenalism
C vitiligo, weakness and hypotension
D increased insulin requirements in diabetic patients
E amenorrhoea and loss of body hair

50
Typical features of secondary adrenocortical insufficiency include
A impaired gonadotrophin secretion usually precedes ACTH deficiency
B impaired plasma cortisol response 30 minutes after ACTH stimulation
C vitiligo and skin hyperpigmentation
D hypotension and hyperkalaemia
E preservation of the normal diurnal rhythm of cortisol secretion

51
In the treatment of primary adrenocortical insufficiency
A when analgesia is required, morphine is the preferred drug
B fludrocortisone is usually unnecessary unless there is hyperkalaemia
C the dose of cortisol should not be increased without medical advice
D adrenal crisis requires intravenous dextrose/saline and hydrocortisone
E typical maintenance therapy comprises at least 50 mg cortisol daily

52
Recognised features of congenital adrenal hyperplasia include
A C21-hydroxylase enzyme deficiency
B decreased plasma cortisol and aldosterone concentrations
C increased mortality in male infants
D tall stature and precocious puberty
E increased plasma 17 alpha-hydroxyprogesterone concentration

Answers
46 C D E
47 B C
48 A B C E
49 A C E

50 A B
51 D
52 A B C D E

53
The insulin-induced hypoglycaemia stimulation test is
A mandatory in the confirmation of secondary hypoadrenalism
B terminated when the plasma glucose falls below 2.2 mmol/L
C contraindicated in ischaemic heart disease and epilepsy
D contraindicated in advanced hypopituitarism
E an unreliable test of hypothalamic function

54
The typical features of phaeochromocytoma include
A predominantly adrenaline rather than noradrenaline secretion
B episodic nausea with sweating and marked skin pallor
C episodic headaches with epigastric/chest pain and palpitation
D episodes of angor animi with hypertension and glycosuria
E control of symptoms following propranolol therapy alone

55
Recognised causes of impotence include
A pituitary microprolactinoma
B psychological distress
C peripheral vascular disease
D diabetes mellitus
E multiple sclerosis

56
In male infertility associated with oligospermia
A increased plasma FSH levels suggest testicular dysfunction
B testicular biopsy should be undertaken to exclude malignancy
C decreased seminal fructose levels suggest seminal vesicle disease
D gonadotrophin therapy usually restores normal fertility
E normal plasma FSH levels suggest obstruction is the cause

57
Hypogonadotrophic hypogonadism is typically associated with
A atrophy of the testicular interstitial (Leydig) cells
B Klinefelter's syndrome (XXY)
C isolated GnRH deficiency (Kallmann's syndrome)
D haemochromatosis
E hepatic cirrhosis

58
The clinical features of male hypogonadism include
A total absence of pubic hair if pre-pubertal in onset
B growth retardation if pre-pubertal in onset
C atrophy of the external genitalia if post-pubertal in onset
D impairment of strength, libido and erectile function
E sweating with hot flushes after post-pubertal castration

59
Recognised causes of hypergonadotrophic hypogonadism include
A Klinefelter's syndrome
B Turner's syndrome
C autoimmune ovarian disease
D syphilis and gonorrhoea
E cryptorchidism

60
In cryptorchidism with inguinal testes
A the individual is usually otherwise normal
B hypogonadotrophic hypogonadism should be excluded
C the seminiferous tubules are typically normal
D testicular interstitial cell function is usually normal
E treatment with chorionic gonadotrophin or GnRH is contraindicated

---

Answers
53 B C D
54 B C D
55 A B C D E
56 A C E

57 C
58 C D E
59 A B C D E
60 A B D

61
Recognised causes of primary amenorrhoea include
A endometriosis
B congenital adrenal hyperplasia
C Turner's syndrome (XO)
D gluten enteropathy
E craniopharyngioma

62
Recognised causes of secondary amenorrhoea include
A pituitary microprolactinoma
B anorexia nervosa
C hydatidiform mole
D arrhenoblastoma
E Stein-Leventhal syndrome

63
The typical features of idiopathic premature menopause include
A decreased plasma LH and FSH concentrations
B hirsutism and clitoral hypertrophy
C bone fractures due to osteomalacia
D superficial dyspareunia and dysuria
E age at onset 45–55 years

64
The following statements about diabetes mellitus are true
A the UK prevalence is approximately 1%
B the disorder is more common in nulliparous than multiparous women
C type I IDDM is typically inherited as an autosomal dominant trait
D type II NIDDM increases in prevalence with advancing age
E hyperglycaemia occurs only after 50% reduction in islet cell mass

65
Type I insulin-dependent diabetes mellitus is associated with
A HLA DR3 and viral initiation of type 1a IDDM in patients aged < 30
B HLA DR4 in females with type 1b IDDM and islet cell antibodies
C serum islet cell antibodies in > 80% of newly-diagnosed patients
D autoimmune disorders and organ-specific antibodies in type 1a IDDM
E serum insulin-binding antibodies in high titre in type 1b IDDM

66
Secondary diabetes mellitus (type II NIDDM) is associated with
A hepatic cirrhosis
B haemochromatosis
C Conn's syndrome (primary hyperaldosteronism)
D pancreatic carcinoma
E thyrotoxicosis, phaeochromocytoma and acromegaly

67
The following statements about type II diabetes mellitus are true
A there is clear evidence of disordered autoimmunity in NIDDM
B both the insulin and the immune response genes are on chromosome 6
C patients with NIDDM typically exhibit hypersensitivity to insulin
D obesity predisposes to NIDDM in genetically-susceptible individuals
E insulin secretion in response to amino acids is normal in NIDDM

68
Biochemical consequences of diabetes mellitus include
A extra-cellular fluid depletion
B decreased glycogenolysis
C decreased lipolysis
D increased gluconeogenesis
E increased urinary excretion of potassium and magnesium

Answers
61 B C D E
62 A B C D E
63 D
64 A D

65 A B C
66 A B D E
67 D E
68 A D E

69
In decompensated diabetes mellitus
A polyuria results from the increased osmolality of the glomerular filtrate
B hyperpnoea is the result of acidosis due to lactic and keto- acids
C water and electrolyte depletion is greater in the mentally confused
D increases in lipolysis reflect the degree of insulin deficiency
E insulin deficiency inhibits the peripheral utilisation of ketoacids

70
The pathological hallmarks of diabetes mellitus include
A cytological signs of residual beta cell hyperactivity in NIDDM
B increased permeability of thickened capillary basement membranes
C impaired insulin secretion in response to glucose stimulation
D beta cell degeneration in patients with IDDM aged < 40 years
E abnormal thickening of basement membranes in all of the capillaries

71
Latent rather than potential diabetes mellitus is suggested by
A an abnormal glucose tolerance test (GTT) developing in pregnancy
B an abnormal GTT returning to normal following weight reduction
C a normal GTT which becomes abnormal during glucocorticoid therapy
D a child with a normal GTT but whose parents both have type I IDDM
E an indentical twin with a normal GTT whose twin has type I IDDM

72
The oral glucose tolerance test
A is described as diabetic if the 2 hour blood glucose > 10 mmol/L
B is described as diabetic if the fasting blood glucose > 6.7 mmol/L
C is undertaken following 3 days of dietary carbohydrate restriction
D is best administered using 75 grams of glucose in 250 ml of water
E is described as diabetic if any blood glucose exceeds 12 mmol/L

73
The following statements about glucose estimations are true
A the plasma glucose is 15% lower than whole blood concentrations
B the urinary dip-stix is glucose-specific
C urinary dip-stix indicates glucose concentrations > 5 mmol/L
D a positive urinary dip-stix in the young usually indicates IDDM
E alimentary glycosuria often heralds the later development of NIDDM

74
Typical presentations of diabetes mellitus include
A weight loss and nocturia
B balanitis or puritus vulvae
C epigastric pain and vomiting
D limb pains with absent ankle reflexes
E increasing myopia and glycosuria

75
In the dietary management of diabetes mellitus
A 60% of patients also require hypoglycaemic drug therapy
B carbohydrate intakes should be 50% of total calorie intake
C ice cream and chocolates should never be consumed
D fat intakes should not exceed 35% of total calorie intake
E in obese patients, calorie intake should not exceed 800 kcal/day

---

Answers
69 A B C D
70 B C D
71 A B C

72 A B D
73 B
74 A B C D E
75 B D

76
Sulphonylurea drug therapy in diabetes mellitus
A causes more weight gain when given with diguanide therapy
B decrease plasma immunoreactive insulin concentrations
C decrease the number of peripheral insulin receptors
D decrease hepatic glycogenolysis and gluconeogenesis
E causes alcohol-induced flushing as a dominantly-inherited trait

77
The following statements about insulin therapy are true
A the duration of action of neutral insulins = 6 hours
B the duration of action of depot insulin = 12 hours +
C insulins are absorbed more rapidly from the leg than the arm
D isophane type insulins do not contain protamine
E human insulins are less potent than animal-derived insulins

78
In the management of a newly-diagnosed 30 year old diabetic
A an experience of insulin-induced hypoglycaemia is mandatory
B insulin requirements during the first 8 weeks often decrease
C insulin should normally be administered once daily initially
D glycosylated haemoglobin levels should be monitored weekly
E during pregnancy, 6-hourly urine testing is recommended

79
Typical symptoms of hypoglycaemia in diabetic patients include
A feelings of faintness and hunger
B tremor, palpitation and dizziness
C headache, diplopia and confusion
D abnormal behaviour despite plasma glucose > 4 mmol/L
E nocturnal sweating, nightmares and convulsions

80
In the treatment of severe hypoglycaemia in diabetic patients
A 50 ml 50% glucose should be given intravenously
B glucagon should not be used if caused by sulphonylureas
C on metformin therapy alone, an alternative explanation is likely
D recovery is invariably complete within an hour of therapy
E hospital admission is usually unnecessary if due to chlorpropamide

81
In the differential diagnosis of diabetic coma features suggesting hypoglycaemia rather than ketoacidosis include
A systemic hypotension
B brisk tendon reflexes
C air hunger
D moist skin and tongue
E abdominal pain

82
The typical clinical features of diabetic ketoacidosis include
A abdominal pain and air hunger
B rapid, weak pulse and hypotension
C profuse sweating and oliguria
D vomiting and constipation
E coma with extensor plantar responses

Answers
76 D E
77 A B
78 A B

79 A B C D E
80 A B C
81 B D
82 A B D

83
Typical findings in diabetic ketoacidosis include
A water deficit of 5–10 litres
B both sodium and potassium deficits of at least 400 mmol
C arterial blood gas analysis PaO_2 7 kPa, $PaCO_2$ 7 kPa and pH = 7.2
D decreased serum potassium concentration at presentation
E peripheral blood leucocytosis

84
In the management of diabetic ketoacidosis
A intracellular water deficit is best restored using normal saline
B potassium should be given irrespective of the serum concentration
C bicarbonate infusion is often only necessary in renal failure
D dextrose should be avoided unless hypoglycaemia supervenes
E acute circulatory failure requires the infusion of dextran or plasma

85
Complications pathognomonic of diabetic microangiopathy include
A nodular glomerulosclerosis
B hard and soft retinal exudates
C mononeuritis multiplex
D rubeosis iridis
E cataracts

86
In the management of diabetes mellitus during pregnancy
A there is a predisposition to hydramnios
B the baby is usually smaller than expected from gestational age
C delivery should be undertaken by Caesarian section at week 36
D mild diabetes responds well to sulphonylurea and diet therapy
E insulin requirements usually decrease throughout pregnancy

87
In the management of diabetics requiring elective surgery
A patients should stop sulphonylureas 24 hours prior to surgery
B insulin should be given preoperatively to prevent ketoacidosis
C patients with NIDDM require insulin cover for major surgery
D sliding-scale insulin therapy is preferrable post-operatively
E glucose-insulin infusion is the optimal method perioperatively

88
In the classification of hyperlipidaemias
A chylomicronaemia is characteristic of types I and V
B hypertriglyceridaemia is associated with types III, IV and V
C hypercholesterolaemia is typical of types II, III, IV
D tendon xanthomata are typical of type IIa hypercholesterolaemia
E palmar xanthomata are characteristic of type III hyperlipidaemia

89
In the treatment of hyperlipidaemia in patients age < 60 years
A dietary fat restriction reduces the plasma cholesterol by 10%
B lowering a plasma cholesterol > 6.5 mmol/L is of no proven value
C drug therapy is usually necessary if plasma cholesterol > 7.8 mmol/L
D high plasma HDL/LDL ratios indicate the need for drug therapy
E fibrates reduce cholesterol synthesis by inhibiting HMG CoA reductase

---

Answers
83 A B E
84 C E
85 A D
86 none

87 A C E
88 A B C D E
89 A C

90
In the classification of acute and non-acute porphyrias
A delta-ALA synthetase activity is increased in all porphyrias
B porphobilinogen deaminase activity is reduced in acute porphyrias
C neuropsychiatric features are typical of the non-acute porphyrias
D photosensitivity is typical of the acute porphyrias
E variegate porphyria and coproporphyria are acute porphyrias

91
The typical features of acute intermittent porphyria include
A increased porphobilinogen deaminase activity
B onset of symptoms rarely occurring before puberty
C vomiting, constipation and abdominal pain
D hypertension and tachycardia
E exacerbation by diamorphine and chlorpromazine therapy

92
The typical features of porphyria cutanea tarda include
A autosomal dominant inheritance
B scleroderma-like thickening of the skin
C hepatomegaly with haemosiderosis
D photosensitivity and diabetes mellitus
E increased urinary porphobilinogen excretion

Answers
90 A B E
91 B C D

92 B C D

Diseases of the Blood

1
In the normal formation of blood cells
A foetal hepatic and splenic haematopoiesis is active until birth
B all lymphocytes originate in the bone marrow
C haematopoiesis in adults extends to the femoral and humeral heads
D the proerythroblast precedes the development of the normoblast
E erythropoietin is produced by renal glomerular mesangial cells

2
Mature erythrocytes
A contain blood group antigens in their cytoplasm
B stain with methylene blue due to ribosomes producing haemoglobin
C derive energy from glucose to fuel the Na^+/K^+ ionic pump
D labelled with ^{51}chromium have a circulation half-life = 120 days
E contain carbonic anhydrase which facilitates the transport of CO_2

3
Haemoglobin
A F comprises two alpha and two delta chains
B A2 comprises two alpha and two gamma chains
C has four porphyrin rings each containing ferrous iron
D is an important buffer of carbonic acid
E oxygen binding is increased by RBC 2-3-diphosphoglycerate

4
Mature neutrophil granulocytes
A comprise > 50% of the total peripheral blood WBC in health
B remain in the circulation for less than 12 hours
C exhibit increased nuclear segmentation in infection
D are derived from a different stem cell to that of monocytes
E produce the vitamin B_{12} binding protein transcobalamin 111

5
Platelets (thrombocytes)
A have a circulation life span of 10 hours in healthy subjects
B are produced and regulated under the control of thrombopoietins
C contain small nuclear remnants called Howell-Jolly bodies
D decrease in number in response to aspirin therapy
E release serotonin and thromboxanes

6
The following statements about RBC morphology are true
A hypochromia is pathognomonic of iron deficiency
B polychromasia indicates active production of new RBCs
C poikilocytosis is invariably associated with anisocytosis
D punctate basophilia is a typical feature of beta-thalassaemia
E target cells are associated with hyposplenism and liver disease

Answers
1 B C D
2 C E
3 C D

4 A B E
5 B E
6 B C D E

7
The following statements about white blood cells are true
A leucopenia in severe pyogenic infection augurs a poor prognosis
B infants often respond to bacterial infection with a lymphocytosis
C monocytosis is a recognised feature of malaria and tuberculosis
D eosinophilia is a characteristic finding in brucellosis
E myelocytes in the peripheral blood are pathognomonic of leukaemia

8
Iron
A content of blood is about 500 mg per litre
B losses in the healthy male are about 3 mg per day
C content of the adult body is about 5 grams
D is usually stored in hepatocytes as haemosiderin
E in the healthy diet amounts to 10–15 mg per day

9
Hypochromic anaemia in childhood is
A more common in breast-fed than bottle-fed infants
B unlikely to be due to gluten enteropathy below the age of 5
C invariably due to iron deficiency
D more difficult to recognise clinically than in adults
E not usually associated with maternal iron deficiency

10
Typical symptoms attributable entirely to anaemia include
A tiredness and malaise
B breathlessness and palpitation
C peripheral paraesthesiae and oedema
D angina and claudication
E tinnitus and dizziness

11
In iron deficiency anaemia
A the tongue is typically painful and heavily furred
B nail brittleness precedes the concavity of koilonychia
C the bone marrow in severe cases exhibits megaloblastosis
D beeturia and in childhood, pica are recognised features
E neurological signs if present are usually due to the anaemia

12
Peripheral blood findings in dietary iron deficiency include
A microcytosis preceding the development of hypochromia
B ovalocytosis, elliptocytosis and polychromasia
C mean corpuscular haemoglobin concentration < 50% of normal
D numerous target cells and Howell-Jolly bodies
E neutrophil leucocyte hypersegmentation and thrombocytosis

13
In the treatment of iron deficiency anaemia with iron
A folic acid should also be given if the anaemia is severe
B iron absorption is only minimally increased in mild anaemia
C inorganic iron compounds are better absorbed than organic iron
D maximal reticulocyte counts usually develop within 7–10 days
E parenteral iron is usually more effective than oral iron

Answers
7 A B C
8 A C
9 A D
10 A B C E

11 B D
12 A B E
13 D

14
Hypochromic microcytic anaemia is a recognised finding in
A haemolytic anaemia
B primary sideroblastic anaemia
C hypothyroidism
D beta-thalassemia
E rheumatoid arthritis

15
Normocytic normochromic anaemia is an expected feature of
A alcoholic liver disease
B chronic renal failure
C hypothyroidism
D kwashiorkor
E scurvy

16
Macrocytic anaemia is a typical finding in
A folic acid deficiency
B haemolytic anaemia
C alcohol abuse
D primary sideroblastic anaemia
E myelodysplastic syndrome

17
Vitamin B$_{12}$ deficiency megaloblastic anaemia typically occurs in
A strict vegetarians
B gluten enteropathy
C Addisonian pernicious anaemia
D jejunal diverticulosis
E ileo-caecal Crohn's disease

18
Typical haematological findings in megaloblastic anaemia include
A pancytopenia and oval macrocytosis
B neutrophil leucocyte hypersegmentation
C anisocytosis and poikilocytosis
D reticulocytosis and polychromasia
E excess urinary urobilinogen and bilirubinuria

19
Folate and vitamin B$_{12}$ deficiency both typically produce
A subacute combined degeneration of the spinal cord
B intermittent glossitis and diarrhoea
C mild jaundice and splenomegaly
D dementia and peripheral neuropathy
E marked weight loss

20
Characteristic features of Addisonian pernicious anaemia include
A onset before the age of 30 years
B gastric parietal cell and intrinsic factor antibodies in the serum
C increased serum bilirubin and lactate dehydrogenase concentrations
D four-fold increase in the risk of developing gastric carcinoma
E Schilling test invariably reverts to normal with intrinsic factor

21
Folate deficiency megaloblastic anaemia typically occurs in
A strict vegetarians
B gluten enteropathy
C pregnancy
D phenytoin therapy
E hookworm infection

Answers
14 B D E
15 B C D E
16 A B C E
17 A C D E

18 A B C
19 B C E
20 B C D
21 B C D

22
Typical features of primary sideroblastic anaemia include
A microcytic hypochromic anaemia
B X-linked mode of inheritance
C partial response to iron therapy
D ring sideroblasts on bone marrow cytology
E progression to acute leukaemia

23
Recognised associations of acquired sideroblastic anaemia include
A macrocytic anaemia
B rheumatoid arthritis
C carcinomatosis
D myelodysplastic syndromes
E pyridoxine deficiency

24
Typical features of the myelodysplastic syndromes include
A presentation before the age of 40 years
B macrocytic anaemia and pancytopenia
C ring sideroblasts present on bone marrow cytology
D clonal chromosomal abnormalities in 50% of patients
E risk of progression to immune deficiency and acute leukaemia

25
Recognised causes of pancytopenia include
A systemic lupus erythematosus
B indomethacin and sulphonamide therapy
C hepatitis A infection
D megaloblastic anaemia
E myelodysplastic syndromes

26
Characteristic features of primary aplastic anaemia include
A peak incidence about the age of 60 years
B normocytic normochromic anaemia with thrombocytosis
C bone marrow trephine is required to confirm the diagnosis
D splenomegaly indicating extramedullary erythropoiesis
E paroxysmal nocturnal haemoglobinuria

27
Indications for bone marrow transplantation include
A aplastic anaemia
B acute myeloblastic leukaemia
C Hodgkin's disease
D chronic myeloid leukaemia
E beta-thalassaemia minor

28
Typical features suggesting intravascular haemolysis include
A bilirubinuria and haemoglobinuria
B methaemalbuminaemia and haemosiderinuria
C increased serum haptoglobin concentration
D increased plasma haemoglobin concentration
E rigors and splenomegaly

29
Laboratory features suggesting haemolytic anaemia include
A increased serum lactate dehydrogenase concentration
B unconjugated hyperbilirubinaemia and excess urobilinogenuria
C peripheral blood neutrophil leucocytosis and reticulocytosis
D peripheral blood polychromasia and macrocytosis
E bone marrow erythroid hyperplasia

Answers
22 A B D
23 A B C D E
24 B C D E
25 A B C D E

26 C E
27 A B D
28 B D E
29 A B C D E

30
Haemolytic anaemia is a recognised complication of
A prosthetic heart valves
B mycoplasmal pneumonia
C megaloblastic anaemia
D malarial infection
E sulphonamide therapy

31
Typical features of hereditary spherocytosis include
A splenomegaly and gallstones
B intravascular haemolysis
C decreased RBC osmotic fragility
D transient aplastic anaemia
E positive Coomb's antiglobulin test

32
Glucose-6-phosphate dehydrogenase (G6PD) deficiency produces
A intravascular haemolysis especially in black Africans
B peripheral blood spherocytosis without anaemia
C an X-linked recessive haemolytic anaemia
D reticulocytosis with Heinz bodies in the red blood cells
E acute haemolysis induced by opiate analgesics

33
The typical clinical features of sickle-cell anaemia include
A haemolytic and aplastic crises
B neonatal spherocytic haemolytic anaemia
C renal papillary, pulmonary and mesenteric infarction
D splenomegaly with hypersplenism
E bone necrosis and Salmonella osteomyelitis

34
Recognised hazards in sickle-cell disease include
A high altitude
B pregnancy
C dehydration
D bloodless field surgery e.g. Bier's block
E hypothermia and infection

35
The typical features of the beta-thalassemias include
A peripheral blood macrocytosis and anaemia
B hepatosplenomegaly and growth retardation
C mongoloid facies with frontal bossing
D neonatal haemolytic anaemia
E leg ulceration and gallstones

36
The typical features of autoimmune haemolytic anaemia include
A peripheral blood spherocytosis and polychromasia
B fever with haemoglobinuria and haemosiderinuria
C association with systemic lupus erythematosus
D positive Coomb's antiglobulin test and splenomegaly
E association with lymphoproliferative disease

37
In isoimmune haemolytic disease of the newborn
A ABO rather than Rhesus incompatibility is usually the more severe
B neonatal jaundice is usually present at birth
C hepatosplenomegaly and peripheral blood normoblasts are common
D the disease decreases in severity with successive pregnancies
E anti-D immunoglobulin prevents the development of maternal antibodies

Answers
30 A B C D E
31 A D
32 A C D
33 A C E

34 A B C D E
35 B C E
36 A B C D E
37 C E

38
Clinical features suggesting an incompatible blood transfusion include
A asymptomatic during the transfusion of the first 250 ml of blood
B rigors, nausea and vomiting
C chest pain and lumbar back pain
D bradycardia with hypertension
E oliguric acute renal failure and haemoglobinuria

39
Recognised causes of an absolute erythrocytosis include
A myelodysplasia
B hepatocellular carcinoma
C chronic pyelonephritis
D obesity and hypertension
E cerebellar haemangioblastoma

40
The typical features of polycythaemia rubra vera include
A predominance in females aged < 40 years
B splenomegaly, leucocytosis and thrombocytosis
C headaches, pruritus and peptic ulcer dyspepsia
D decreased leucocyte alkaline phosphatase score
E increased blood viscosity associated with vascular disease

41
Recognised causes of neutropenia and agranulocytosis include
A folic acid deficiency
B sulphasalazine therapy
C sickle-cell anaemia
D infectious mononucleosis
E carbimazole therapy

42
Peripheral blood monocytosis is a recognised finding in
A glandular fever and brucellosis
B infective endocarditis
C rheumatoid arthritis
D Crohn's disease and ulcerative colitis
E carcinomatosis

43
Peripheral blood lymphocytosis is an expected finding in
A typhoid fever
B pneumococcal pneumonia
C measles and rubella
D Hodgkin's disease
E chronic lymphatic leukaemia

44
Peripheral blood neutrophil leucocytosis is an expected finding in
A connective tissue disease
B corticosteroid therapy
C pregnancy
D whooping cough
E mesenteric infarction

45
Recognised causes of leucoerythroblastic anaemia include
A carcinomatosis
B miliary tuberculosis
C myelofibrosis
D whooping cough
E severe bleeding or haemolysis

Answers
38 B C E
39 B E
40 B C E
41 A B E

42 A B C D E
43 A C E
44 A B C E
45 A B C E

46
Typical clinical features of infectious mononucleosis include
A incubation period of 7–10 days
B sore throat, dysphagia and headache
C right hypochondrial tenderness
D Epstein Barr virus IgM antibodies
E erythromycin-induced skin rash

47
Characteristic features of acute leukaemia include
A rapid onset of fever and anaemia
B mouth ulceration and gingival hypertrophy
C myalgia, arthralgia and skin rashes
D microcytic anaemia and leucopenia
E hypocellular bone marrow cytology

48
Acute lymphoblastic leukaemia
A usually develops in patients > 20 years old
B typically produces blast cell cytoplasmic Auer rods
C responds better to chemotherapy than other acute leukaemias
D is the most common of all acute leukaemias
E is a typical complication of myelomatosis

49
Clinical features of chronic myeloid leukaemia (CML) include
A painful splenomegaly and priapism
B sternal tenderness, gout and arthralgia
C generalised lymphadenopathy
D tendency to bleeding and gout
E median survival of 10 years with chemotherapy

50
Laboratory findings in chronic myeloid leukaemia include
A leucoerythroblastic anaemia and thrombocytosis
B peripheral blood neutrophilia, eosinophilia and basophilia
C chromosomal translocation 22q – /9q + in 90% of patients
D increased neutrophil leucocyte alkaline phosphatase score
E transformation to acute lymphoblastic leukaemia

51
Typical features of chronic lymphatic leukaemia include
A onset in younger patients than in CML
B development of autoimmune haemolytic anaemia
C presentation with massive hepatosplenomegaly and anaemia
D lymphadenopathy associated with recurrent infections
E median survival of 10 years following chemotherapy

52
The laboratory features in chronic lymphatic leukaemia include
A hyperuricaemia and thrombocytosis
B folic acid deficiency and hypogammaglobulinaemia
C peripheral blood lymphocytosis in the absense of lymphoblasts
D positive Coomb's test and Bence-Jones proteinuria
E transformation to acute leukaemia is more common than in CML

53
The presence of lymphadenopathy and splenomegaly is typical in
A myelomatosis
B chronic lymphatic leukaemia
C chronic myeloid leukaemia
D infectious mononucleosis
E myelofibrosis

Answers
46 A B C D
47 A B C
48 C
49 A B D

50 A C E
51 B D
52 B C D
53 B D

54
The typical features of myelofibrosis include
A absence of splenomegaly or lymphadenopathy
B leucoerythroblastic blood film with tear-drop poikilocytes
C increased leucocyte neutrophil alkaline phosphatase score
D folic acid deficiency and hyperuricaemia
E absent bone marrow megakaryocytes and thrombocytopenia

55
Recognised clinical features of myelomatosis include
A peak incidence between the ages 60–70 years
B amyloidosis with Bence-Jones proteinuria
C median survival of 2 years despite chemotherapy
D recurrent infections and pancytopenia
E increased serum calcium, urate and blood viscosity

56
In the differential diagnosis of myelomatosis from benign monoclonal gammopathy, the following features favour myeloma
A monoclonal gammopathy with normal serum immunoglobulin levels
B bone marrow plasmacytosis > 20%
C lymphadenopathy and splenomegaly
D Bence-Jones proteinuria
E multiple osteolytic lesions on X-ray

57
Following rehydration, a poor prognosis in myelomatosis is suggested by the presence of
A blood urea > 10 mmol/L
B decreased $beta_2$ – microglobulin concentration
C blood haemoglobin < 8 grams/dL
D Bence-Jones proteinuria
E renal amyloidosis

58
Typical histopathological features of Hodgkin's disease include
A Reed-Sternberg binucleate giant cells and lymphocytes
B increased tissue eosinophils, neutrophils and plasma cells
C increased fibrous stroma in the nodular sclerosing type
D frequent involvement of the central nervous system
E splenic involvement is rare in the absence of splenomegaly

59
The clinical features of Hodgkin's disease include
A painless cervical lymphadenopathy
B anaemia typically indicating bone marrow involvement
C impaired T cell function in the absence of lymphopenia
D pruritus and alcohol-induced abdominal pain
E overall 10 year survival > 60% following treatment

60
In the Ann Arbor staging of lymphomas
A intra-thoracic and intra-abdominal lymphadenopathy = stage III
B splenomegaly and intra-abdominal lymphadenopathy = stage IIIS
C diffuse hepatic or bone marrow involvement = stage IV
D gastric and splenic involvement = IISE
E pulmonary hilar lymphadenopathy with fever = stage IB

Answers
54 B C D
55 A B C D E
56 B D E
57 A C E

58 A B C
59 A C D E
60 A C D E

61
Typical characteristics of non-Hodgkin's lymphoma include
A follicular cell histology indicating a low grade lymphoma
B bone marrow and splenic involvement are present from the onset
C involvement of the stomach and thyroid gland is common
D the majority are T cell rather than B cell in origin
E better prognosis in high grade rather than low grade lymphomas

62
Normal platelets contain the following haemostatic factors
A serotonin
B beta-thromboglobulin
C factor V
D fibrinogen
E ristocetin co-factor (factor VIII-von Willebrand factor)

63
Haemostatic factors circulating in the blood include
A thromboplastin
B fibrin
C factor VIII
D factor IX
E plasminogen

64
Prolongation of the prothrombin time is typical in
A fibrinogen deficiency
B factor X deficiency
C factor VII deficiency
D factor V deficiency
E factor II deficiency

65
Prolongation of the partial thromboplastin time is typical in
A factor I or II deficiency
B factor VII deficiency
C factor VIII or X deficiency
D factor XIII deficiency
E factor XII, XI or IX deficiency

66
Vitamin K deficiency and oral anticoagulant therapy both produce
A factor V deficiency
B factor II and VII deficiency
C factor IX and X deficiency
D prolongation of the thrombin and the prothrombin times
E prolongation of the partial thromboplastin and prothrombin times

67
Coagulopathies associated with liver failure include
A thrombocytopenia and thrombasthenia
B prolongation of the partial thromboplastin time
C prolongation of the thrombin and prothrombin times
D impaired synthesis of factors I, II, V, VII, IX and X
E impaired synthesis of factor VIII

68
Disseminated intravascular coagulation is a complication of
A amniotic fluid embolism
B incompatible blood transfusion
C hypovolaemic and anaphylactic shock
D septicaemic shock
E carcinomatosis

Answers
61 A B C
62 A B C D E
63 C D E
64 B C D E

65 A C E
66 B C E
67 A B C D
68 A B C D E

69
Features of disseminated intravascular coagulation include
A thrombocytopenia
B burr cells and schistocytes in the peripheral blood
C decreased serum fibrin degradation products
D normal prothrombin time and normal thrombin time
E prolongation of the partial thromboplastin time

70
The bleeding time is characteristically prolonged in
A ascorbic acid deficiency
B thrombocytopenia
C haemophilia
D warfarin therapy
E von Willebrand's disease

71
Haemorrhagic disorders due to decreased clotting factors include
A hereditary haemorrhagic telangiectasia
B Christmas disease
C senile purpura
D Henoch-Schonlein purpura
E haemophilia

72
The following statements about severe haemophilia A are true
A the disorder is transmitted in an X-linked recessive mode
B recurrent haemarthroses and haematuria are typical features
C both partial thromboplastin and prothrombin times are prolonged
D factor VIII has a biological half-life = 8 days
E desmopressin (DDAVP) significantly increases factor VIII levels

73
The typical features of von Willebrand's disease include
A an X-linked recessive mode of inheritance
B prolongation of the bleeding and partial thromboplastin times
C recurrent severe haemarthroses and thrombocytopenia
D impaired ristocetin-induced platelet aggregation
E clinical response to fibrinolytic inhibitors

74
Haemorrhagic disorders due to defective blood vessels include
A anaphylactoid purpura
B ascorbic acid deficiency
C septicaemia
D Christmas disease
E uraemia

75
Recognised causes of thrombocytosis include
A myeloproliferative disorders
B iron deficiency anaemia
C hypersplenism
D carcinomatosis
E connective tissue disorders

76
Recognised causes of thrombocytopenia include
A megaloblastic anaemia
B acquired immunodeficiency syndrome
C disseminated intravascular coagulation
D von Willebrand's disease
E aspirin, thiazide and sulphonamide therapy

Answers
69 A B E
70 B E
71 B E
72 A B

73 B D E
74 A B C E
75 A B D E
76 A B C E

77
Typical features of idiopathic thrombocytopenic purpura include
A IgG-mediated thrombocytopenia
B predominantly affects patients > 40 years old
C prolongation of the bleeding time
D palpable splenomegaly
E response to corticosteroid therapy

78
Hypercoagulation abnormalities are a recognised feature of
A the lupus anticoagulant (cardiolipin antibody) in SLE
B congenital deficiency of anti-thrombin III
C Waldenstrom's macroglobulinaemia
D polycythaemia rubra vera
E chronic myeloid leukaemia

Answers
77 A C E
78 A B C D E

Diseases of connective tissues, joints and bones

1
Spinal scoliosis
A in childhood is a normal finding until the age of 3 years old
B if postural in origin, disappears on spinal flexion
C if attributable to pain, is associated with limited spinal flexion
D if structural in origin, persists on spinal flexion
E is a typical feature of fixed adduction deformity of the hip

2
Lordosis of the lumbar spine
A in childhood typically appears before the child begins to walk
B decreases during pregnancy
C is more often apparent in adults than in children
D when extreme is usually termed gibbus
E increases in degenerative lumbar disc disease

3
The following statements about joint deformities are true
A talipes deformity indicates ankle plantar flexion with adduction
B in genu varus the knee deviates towards the midline
C cubitus varus is typical of the normal female elbow
D lordosis of the cervical spine is termed torticollis
E angular kyphosis of the thoracic spine is termed gibbus

4
The gait of a patient with
A a painful knee is typified by an abnormal rhythm
B hip ankylosis without deformity is usually normal
C hemiplegia is characterised by an outward swing of the limb
D myopathy of the gluteal muscles is typically waddling
E bilateral foot drop is characteristically high-stepping

5
The following statements about musculoskeletal pains are true
A the pain of inflammatory arthritis is typically worse by day
B the pain of ligamentous strain is usually only felt on movement
C the pain of impacted fractures is invariably worse on movement
D muscle pain is typically unaffected by isometric contraction
E the pain of osteoarthrosis is typically worse on resting

6
The following hand muscles are innervated as described below
A flexor pollicis brevis — ulnar nerve
B adductor pollicis — median nerve
C extensor digitorum longus — radial nerve
D opponens pollicis — median nerve
E all the lumbricals — ulnar nerve

Answers
1 B C D E
2 none
3 E

4 A B C D E
5 none
6 C D

7
Shoulder pain is a recognised feature of
A myocardial ischaemia
B supraspinatus tendonitis
C bronchial carcinoma
D pneumococcal pneumonia
E cervical spondylosis

8
Rotator cuff disorders of the shoulder typically produce
A inability to maintain abduction of the arm to 90 degrees
B inability to shrug the shoulders
C shoulder pain during abduction of the arm
D shoulder pain during isometric contraction of biceps
E recurrent shoulder dislocation

9
The cervical spine is
A typically affected by osteoporotic vertebral collapse
B more liable to dislocation in extension than flexion injuries
C the most mobile section of the vertebral column
D normally lordotic
E characteristically susceptible to disc protrusion

10
The thoracic spine is
A the commonest site of symptomatic disc protrusion
B more mobile in rotation than flexion and extension
C normally lordotic
D typically straight in spinal osteoporosis
E usually scoliotic if affected in poliomyelitis

11
The following statements about the lumbar spine disease are true
A the spinal cord normally terminates at the level of LV4
B the pain of psoas abscess is exacerbated by passive hip flexion
C the lumbar spine is the commonest site of congenital anomalies
D pus from vertebral osteomyelitis usually emerges posteriorly
E backache is an invariable feature if neurological signs develop

12
In lumbar intervertebral disc protrusion syndromes
A impaired straight leg raising suggests an L2/L3 disc prolapse
B femoral nerve root entrapment is exacerbated by hip extension
C inability to lie prone suggests L2/L3 disc prolapse
D scoliosis is typically concave to the side of the disc prolapse
E buttock pain on coughing suggests L3/L4 disc prolapse

13
Dislocation of the hip
A in infants typically occurs when the hip is extended and adducted
B in adults is usually the result of a congenital anomaly
C in adults is more likely to occur when the hip is flexed
D posteriorly produces abduction and external rotation of the leg
E anteriorly produces adduction and internal rotation of the leg

Answers
7 A B C D E
8 C D
9 C D E
10 E

11 C
12 B C D E
13 A C

14
The features of unilateral congenital hip dislocation include
A internal rotation of the limb
B apparent lengthening of the limb
C asymmetry of the thigh and buttock skin folds
D limitation of hip abduction
E limitation of hip flexion

15
On examination of the knee joint
A a small effusion is usually detected by a patellar tap
B collateral ligaments are best assessed with the knee extended
C cruciate ligaments are best assessed with the knee flexed
D crepitus is a typical feature of intra-articular loose bodies
E bruising of one side of the knee suggests cartilage damage

16
Typical features of rupture of the Achilles tendon include
A a palpable gap in the tendon
B absence of plantar flexion of the foot on squeezing the calf
C absence of active plantar flexion of the foot
D inability to stand on tiptoe on the affected foot
E decreased passive dorsiflexion of the foot

17
The typical features of rheumatoid arthritis (RA) include
A onset usually before the age of 30 years
B UK prevalence of 3% with a female-male ratio of 3:1
C association with HLA–D4 and HLA–DR4
D progression to bone and cartilage destruction
E progression to severe disability in 33% of patients

18
Characteristic changes in rheumatoid arthritis include
A diffuse necrotising vasculitis
B increased synovial fluid complement concentration
C subcutaneous nodules with numerous giant cells
D generalised hyperplastic lymphadenopathy
E progression to amyloidosis

19
Typical features of active rheumatoid arthritis include
A fever and weight loss
B macrocytic anaemia
C anterior uveitis
D hypoalbuminaemia
E lymphadenopathy

20
The typical pattern of synovial disease in RA includes
A early involvement of the sacro-iliac joints
B symmetrical peripheral joint involvement
C spindling of the fingers and broadening of the forefeet
D distal interphalangeal joint involvement of fingers and toes
E acromioclavicular and sternoclavicular joint involvement

21
Extra-articular manifestations of rheumatoid arthritis include
A cutaneous ulceration
B pericardial and pleural effusions
C amyloidosis
D peripheral neuropathy
E hypersplenism

Answers
14 C D
15 B C
16 A B D
17 B C D E

18 A D E
19 A D
20 B C E
21 A B C D E

22
The following statements about rheumatoid arthritis are true
A joint pain and stiffness is typically aggravated by rest
B the Rose-Waaler test is positive in about 70% of patients
C joint involvement is additive rather than flitting
D associated scleromalacia typically produces painful red eyes
E Raynaud's and sicca syndrome suggest an alternative diagnosis

23
In the treatment of rheumatoid arthritis
A bed rest accelerates the development of bony ankylosis
B splinting of the affected joints reduces pain and swelling
C physiotheraphy is necessary to avoid flexion contractures
D systemic corticosteroids are contraindicated
E non-steroidal anti-inflammatory drugs retard disease progression

24
Drugs which retard disease progression in RA include
A sulphasalazine
B corticosteroids
C D-penicillamine
D sodium aurothiomalate
E azathioprine

25
A poorer prognosis in rheumatoid arthritis is associated with
A insidious onset of rheumatoid arthritis
B positive rheumatoid factor early in the course of the disease
C early development of subcutaneous nodules and erosive arthritis
D extra-articular manifestations of the disease
E onset with palindromic rheumatism

26
Characteristic features of Sjogren's syndrome include
A Raynaud's phenomenon and hair loss
B dry eyes, mouth and vagina
C hepatosplenomegaly
D renal tubular acidosis and glomerulonephritis
E diffuse interstitial pulmonary fibrosis

27
Typical features of seronegative spondyloarthritis include
A asymmetrical oligoarthritis
B sacro-iliitis and spondylitis
C enthesitis of tendinous insertions
D scleritis and episcleritis
E mitral valve disease

28
Features associated with ankylosing spondylitis include
A peak onset in the second and third decades
B chronic prostatitis
C HLA–B27 in > 90% of affected patients
D faecal carriage of specific Klebsiella enterobacteria
E family history of psoriatic arthritis and Reiter's syndrome

29
Clinical features of ankylosing spondylitis include
A acute anterior uveitis
B aortic incompetence
C atlanto-axial subluxation
D amyloidosis
E apical pulmonary fibrosis

Answers
22 A B C
23 B C
24 A C D E
25 A B C D

26 A B C D E
27 A B C
28 A B C D E
29 A B C D E

30
Features suggesting ankylosing spondylitis include
A early morning low back pain radiating to the buttocks
B persistence of lumbar lordosis on spinal flexion
C chest pain aggravated by breathing
D 'squaring' of the lumbar vertebrae on X-ray
E erosions of the symphysis pubis on X-ray

31
In the treatment of ankylosing spondylitis
A systemic corticosteroid therapy is contraindicated
B prolonged bed rest accelerates functional recovery
C spinal radiotherapy modifies the course of the disease
D spinal deformity is minimised with physiotherapy
E hip joint involvement augurs a poorer prognosis

32
The typical features of Reiter's disease include
A anterior uveitis more often than conjunctivitis
B non-specific urethritis and prostatitis
C symmetrical small joint polyarthritis
D onset 1–3 weeks following bacterial dysentery
E keratoderma blenorrhagica and nail dystrophy

33
Recognised features of Reiter's disease include
A tetracycline therapy prevents progressive arthritis
B sacro-iliitis and spondylitis develops in 15% of patients
C pericarditis, pleurisy and meningo-encephalitis
D fever, weight loss and calcaneal spurs on X-ray
E peripheral blood pancytopenia and elevated ESR

34
Psoriatic arthritis
A is invariably preceded by the development of psoriasis
B affects 25% of patients with psoriasis
C is more common than rheumatoid arthritis especially in females
D has a poorer prognosis than does rheumatoid arthritis
E responds to hydroxochloroquine and D-penicillamine therapy

35
Recognised patterns of psoriatic arthritis include
A asymmetrical oligoarthritis of the fingers and toes
B distal interphalangeal joint involvement with nail dystrophy
C sacro-iliitis and spondylitis
D rheumatoid-like symmetrical small joint arthritis
E arthritis mutilans with telescoping of the digits

36
Diseases associated with sero-negative spondyloarthritis include
A Sjogren's syndrome
B Whipple's disease
C coeliac disease
D ulcerative colitis
E Behcet's disease

Answers
30 A B C D E
31 D E
32 B D E

33 B C D
34 none
35 A B C D E
36 B D E

37
Arthritis in childhood is a typical feature of
A mumps and rubella virus infections
B rheumatic fever
C acute leukaemia
D Henoch Schonlein purpura
E meningococcal infection

38
The following statements about juvenile chronic arthritis are true
A Still's disease usually presents with an unexplained arthritis
B seropositive polyarthritis resembles adult rheumatoid arthritis
C pauciarticular disease in girls is a marker for chronic iritis
D pauciarticular disease in boys resembles ankylosing spondylitis
E seronegative polyarthritis rarely involves the neck or mandible

39
The typical features of Still's disease include
A systemic onset with marked fever and an evanescent rash
B lymphadenopathy and hepatosplenomegaly
C high titres of rheumatoid factor in the serum
D pleurisy, pericarditis and subcutaneous nodules
E progression to arthritis of the neck, wrists, knees and ankles

40
The typical features of rheumatic fever include
A fever with abdominal pain, vomiting and pancarditis
B additive more often than flitting large joint polyarthritis
C onset within 7 days of beta-haemolytic streptococcal infection
D erythema marginatum of the trunk but not the face
E onset usually before the age of 4 years

41
The following statements about infective arthritis are true
A the onset is typically insidious
B preexisting arthritis is a recognised predisposing factor
C small peripheral joints are the most often involved
D salmonella infection is common in sickle cell anaemia
E joint aspiration should be avoided given the risk of septicaemia

42
The typical features of gonoccocal arthritis include
A predominance of young males
B pustular or vesicular rashes
C tenosynovitis and asymmetrical oligoarthritis
D the diagnosis is best established by synovial fluid culture
E residual joint damage is likely

43
The following disorders produce an arthritis as described below
A Lyme disease — relapsing pauciarticular large joint arthritis
B acromegaly — small joint arthritis and hypertrophic spondylosis
C hyperlipidaemia — asymmetrical arthritis of the knees and hips
D chronic sarcoidosis — symmetrical arthritis of the ankles and knees
E amyloidosis — symmetrical small joint arthritis resembling RA

Answers
37 A B C D E
38 B C D
39 A B D E
40 A B D

41 B D
42 B C D
43 A B E

44
Typical features of systemic lupus erythematosus (SLE) include
A commoner in caucasian than black women
B onset is usually in the fourth and fifth decades
C impaired function of suppressor T lymphocytes
D increased prevalence of HLA–B8 and HLA–DR3
E increased serum complement concentrations

45
Characteristic clinical features of SLE include
A Raynaud's phenomenon and photosensitivity
B alopecia and livedo reticularis
C erosive asymmetrical large joint arthritis
D fibrosing alveolitis and glomerulonephritis
E pericarditis and endocarditis

46
Complications of systemic lupus erythematosus include
A transverse myelitis
B depressive psychosis
C peripheral neuropathy
D pancreatitis and cholecystitis
E autoimmune haemolytic anaemia

47
Typical blood findings in systemic lupus erythematosus include
A leucocytosis and thrombocytosis
B impaired coagulation due to anticardiolipin antibodies
C anti-DNA and rheumatoid factor antibodies in high titre
D elevated total haemolytic, C3 and C4 complement levels
E dermoepidermal immune complexes in 'normal' skin biopsies

48
Drug-induced SLE is a recognised feature of treatment with
A aspirin
B hydralazine
C oestrogens
D phenytoin
E phenothiazine

49
The following therapies are helpful in the treatment of SLE
A aspirin-like drugs
B 'pulse' therapy with methylprednisolone
C plasmapheresis
D hydroxychloroquine
E corticosteroids and azathioprine

50
Typical features of mixed connective tissue disease (MCTD) include
A dermatomyositis and polymyositis
B Raynaud's phenomenon and fibrosing alveolitis
C anti-RNA antibodies in high titre
D renal and neurological involvement
E erosive small joint arthritis

51
The clinical features of progressive systemic sclerosis include
A Raynaud's phenomenon and cutaneous telangiectasia
B reflux oesophagitis, dysphagia and colonic dilatation
C fibrosing alveolitis and glomerulonephritis
D peripheral arthritis with 'sausage' swelling of the fingers
E anti-DNA antibodies and decreased serum complement levels

Answers
44 C D
45 A B D E
46 A B C D E
47 B C E

48 B C D E
49 A B C D E
50 A B C
51 A B C D

52
The typical features of polymyositis and dermatomyositis include
A association with HLA–B8, HLA–DR3 and antinuclear antibodies
B proximal muscle weakness with high serum creatine phosphokinase
C erosive asymmetrical large joint arthritis of the lower limbs
D underlying malignancy is usually present if weight loss is marked
E erythematous rash on the knuckles, elbows, knees and face

53
The characteristic features of polymyalgia rheumatica include
A predominantly affects females > 60 years of age
B abrupt onset of neck, back and limb girdle pain and stiffness
C absence of sternoclavicular or acromioclavicular joint tenderness
D muscle tenderness often associated with proximal muscle atrophy
E weight loss with normochromic anaemia and grossly elevated ESR

54
In polymyagia rheumatica
A antinuclear and rheumatoid factor antibodies are often present
B temporal artery biopsy is necessary to confirm the diagnosis
C response to oral corticosteroids typically occurs within 7 days
D corticosteroid therapy should be withdrawn after 6 months
E sudden uniocular blindness suggests steroid-induced cataract

55
Factors predisposing to hyperuricaemia and gout include
A hypothyroidism
B hyperparathyroidism
C chronic lead poisoning
D myeloproliferative disorders
E pyrazinamide and thiazide therapy

56
Recognised clinical features of gout include
A increased urate production in most patients
B cellulitis, tenosynovitis and bursitis
C abrupt onset of severe joint pain and tenderness
D fever and leucocytosis associated with polyarthritis
E acute renal failure in the absence of arthritis

57
In the treatment of acute gout
A indomethacin acts by increasing urinary urate excretion
B colchicine acts by inhibiting leucocyte migration into the joint
C allopurinol acts by inhibiting xanthine oxidase urate production
D probenecid acts by inhibiting renal tubular urate reabsorption
E allopurinol or probenecid should be given within 24 hours of onset

58
Factors predisposing to chondrocalcinosis and pseudo-gout include
A hyperparathyroidism
B haemochromatosis
C hypothyroidism
D hypomagnesaemia
E hypophosphataemia

59
Recognised clinical features of pseudo-gout include
A abrupt onset of a painful swollen knee
B rheumatoid-like small joint arthritis
C osteoarthrosis-like arthritis of the wrists and MCP joints
D absence of efficacy of indomethacin and colchicine
E strongly-negative birefringent joint crystals on microscopy

Answers
52 A B E
53 A B E
54 C
55 A B C D E

56 B C D E
57 B C D
58 A B C D E
59 A B C

60
The clinical features of primary nodal osteoarthrosis include
A joint pain aggravated by rest and relieved by activity
B proximal interphalangeal and MCP joint involvement
C involvement of the hip, knee and spinal apophyseal joints
D strong family history of Heberden's nodes
E microfractures of cartilage and subchondral bone

61
Recognised causes of secondary osteoarthrosis include
A rheumatoid arthritis
B sickle cell anaemia
C hypermobility syndromes
D ochronosis
E chondrocalcinosis

62
Typical features of Paget's disease of bone include
A onset before the age of 50 years
B increased serum alkaline phosphatase and urinary hydroxyproline
C involvement of the skull, spine, femora, tibia and pelvis
D decreased osteoblastic activity with delayed healing of fractures
E risk of development of osteogenic sarcoma

63
Tumours that frequently metastasise to bone include
A colonic carcinoma
B bronchial carcinoma
C prostatic carcinoma
D breast carcinoma
E thyroid carcinoma

64
Typical features of primary osteosarcomas include
A onset before the age of 20 years
B most often develop at the lower end of the tibia
C presentation with pulmonary metastases
D 'sun-ray' appearance on X-ray due to new bone formation
E 5-year survival rates are usually < 10% despite amputation

65
Typical features of chondosarcoma include
A onset before the age of 10 years
B most often develop in the long bones, pelvis and scapulae
C presentation with pain and swelling
D 'onion skin' appearance on X-ray due to periosteal new bone
E 5-year survival rates are better than 50% with surgical resection

66
Typical features of Ewing's sarcoma include
A onset between the ages 5–15 years
B origin in the bone marrow endothelium
C presentation with features suggesting osteomyelitis
D characteristic 'onion skin' appearance on X-ray
E 5-year survival rates are virtually nil despite amputation

67
Typical clinical features of osteomyelitis include
A onset in the sixth and seventh decade
B fever, joint effusion and bone pain
C onset of X-ray changes preceded by an abnormal isotope bone scan
D most often due to Salmonella infection in sickle cell anaemia
E sparing of the disc space in vertebral osteomyelitis

Answers
60 C D E
61 A B C D E
62 B C E
63 B C D E

64 A D E
65 B C E
66 A B C D E
67 B C D

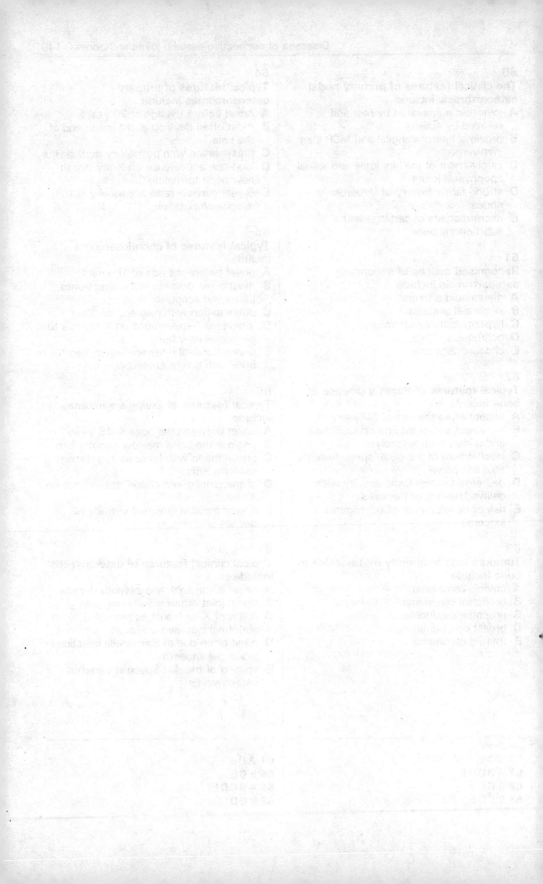

Diseases of the nervous system

1
The following definitions are true
A dysarthria — inability to write
B dysphasia — inability to comprehend or produce speech
C dysphonia — inability to enunciate words clearly
D dyslexia — inability to read
E dysgraphia — inability to interpret visual data

2
Dysphonia is an expected consequence of
A myasthenia gravis
B supranuclear bulbar palsy
C Parkinson's disease
D cerebellar disease
E lesion of Broca's area

3
Dysarthria is an expected consequence of
A bilateral recurrent laryngeal nerve palsies
B supranuclear bulbar palsy
C cerebellar disease
D myasthenia gravis
E lesion of Wernicke's area

4
The speech area of the brain
A includes the superior temporal gyrus
B includes the inferior frontal gyrus
C is in the dominant hemisphere
D in left-handed subjects, is usually in the right hemisphere
E includes the superior parietal lobule of the cerebral cortex

5
The following statements about dyspraxia are true
A it is defined as the inability to coordinate simple movements
B it is readily distinguishable from conversion hysteria
C it is frequently associated with dysphasia
D it is best demonstrated using the finger-nose test
E it is a feature of disease of one or other parietal lobe

6
The following statements about anosmia are true
A it is often described by the patient as loss of taste
B when suspected, it is best confirmed by testing with vinegar
C it is usually the result of neurological disease
D head injury is the commonest neurological cause
E it is a recognised feature of intracranial tumour

7
Typical features of myasthenia gravis include
A absent pupillary reflexes
B motor dysphasia
C ptosis
D muscle wasting
E improvement with i.v. edrophonium

Answers
 1 B D
 2 A B C
 3 B C D
 4 A B C

 5 C
 6 A D E
 7 C E

8
Typical features of Parkinsonism include
A ataxic gait
B nystagmus
C cogwheel rigidity
D festinant gait
E failure to swing the arms while walking

9
Typical findings in cerebellar disease include
A dysmetria
B dysarthria
C intention tremor
D increased muscle tone
E pendular nystagmus

10
Right homonymous hemianopia usually results from damage to
A the left optic tract
B the left optic radiation
C the optic chiasma
D the left lateral geniculate body
E the left optic nerve

11
Conjugate deviation of the eyes is controlled by
A the frontal lobe
B the occipital lobe
C the parabducens nucleus of the pons
D the superior rectus muscle of the adducting eye
E the medial longitudinal bundle

12
Features suggesting a third cranial nerve palsy include
A paralysis of abduction
B absence of facial sweating
C complete ptosis
D pupillary dilatation
E absence of the accommodation reflex

13
Paralysis of the fourth cranial nerve produces
A weakness of the inferior oblique muscle
B impaired upward gaze in abduction
C impaired downward gaze in adduction
D elevation and abduction of the eye
E uniocular nystagmus of the abducted eye

14
Structures traversing the cavernous sinus include
A the mandibular division of the fifth cranial nerve
B the oculomotor nerve
C the trochlear nerve
D the abducent nerve
E the optic nerve

15
Paralysis of the sixth cranial nerve
A produces impaired adduction of the eye
B produces elevation and adduction of the eye
C is a characteristic feature of Wernicke's encephalopathy
D results from disease of the upper pons
E is a recognised feature of posterior fossa tumour

Answers
 8 C D E
 9 A B C
10 A B D
11 A B C E

12 C D E
13 C D
14 B C D
15 C D E

16
The cervical sympathetic outflow
A supplies the sweat glands of the skin of the face
B leaves the spinal cord via the thoracic roots T1–T3
C supplies the levator palpebrae superioris
D supplies the sphincter pupillae
E supplies the muscle which holds the eye forward in the orbit

17
Drooping of the upper eyelid results from a lesion of the
A levator palpebrae superioris
B third cranial nerve
C cervical sympathetic outflow
D seventh cranial nerve
E parabducens nucleus

18
Normal abduction of the right eye with impaired adduction of the left eye on right lateral gaze occurs in lesions of the
A left superior rectus muscle
B left medial rectus muscle
C medial longitudinal bundle
D left sixth cranial nerve
E cerebellum

19
Diplopia on right lateral upward gaze occurs in lesions of the
A left inferior rectus muscle
B right superior rectus muscle
C right lateral rectus muscle
D left inferior oblique muscle
E right superior oblique muscle

20
Absence of pupillary constriction in either eye on shining a light into the right pupil is typical of the following lesions
A bilateral Argyll Robertson pupils
B bilateral Holmes-Adie pupils
C right optic nerve lesion
D right oculomotor nerve lesion
E bilateral chronic iritis

21
On right lateral gaze, unilateral nystagmus of the abducted right eye with impaired adduction of the left eye suggests
A defective left macular vision
B left vestibular neuronitis
C left cerebellar hemisphere disease
D disease of the left medulla oblongata
E disease of the medial longitudinal bundle

22
Recognised causes of impaired facial sensation include
A cavernous sinus disease
B trigeminal neuralgia
C acoustic neuroma
D lesion of the posterior limb of the internal capsule
E lesion of the upper cervical cord segments

23
The spinal (descending) tract of the fifth cranial nerve
A descends to the fifth cervical cord segment
B conducts motor fibres to the lateral pterygoid muscles
C contains pain and temperature nerve fibres from the face
D conveys proprioceptive impulses from the head and neck
E maintains the separation of nerve fibres from the three trigeminal nerve branches

---

Answers
16 A B E
17 A B C
18 B C
19 B C D

20 A B C E
21 E
22 A C D E
23 C

24
Features of an upper motor neurone facial weakness include
A preservation of emotional smiling
B ptosis
C drooping of the angle of the mouth
D inability to wrinkle the forehead
E weakness of the masseter muscle

25
Features of an intracranial lower motor neurone lesion of the facial nerve include
A inability to wrinkle the forehead
B presence of a 'snout' reflex
C upward deviation of the eye on attempted eyelid closure
D deafness due to loss of the nerve to the stapedius muscle
E loss of taste over the anterior two-thirds of the tongue

26
Deafness of the right ear associated with a normal Rinne's test and Weber's test lateralised to the left is compatible with
A Meniere's disease
B presbyacusis
C auditory meatal obstruction
D acoustic neuroma
E otitis media

27
Characteristic features of pseudo-bulbar palsy include
A dysarthria
B dysphagia
C emotional lability
D wasting and fasciculation of the tongue
E absence of the jaw jerk

28
The following statements about muscle fasciculation are true
A it is the spontaneous contraction of single muscle fibres
B it invariably implies the presence of serious disease
C it indicates upper rather than lower motor neurone involvement
D it is invariably accompanied by muscle wasting
E it rarely if ever involves the tongue

29
Upper motor neurone involvement is characterised by
A extensor plantar responses
B absent abdominal reflexes
C absent cremasteric reflexes
D increased muscle tone and tendon reflexes
E plantar flexion of the great toe in response to rapid dorsiflexion of the toes (Rossolimo's sign)

30
Lower motor neurone involvement is characterised by
A flaccid muscle tone
B the rapid onset of muscle wasting
C absent or decreased tendon reflexes
D muscle contractures
E muscle fasciculation

31
Recognised features of extrapyramidal tract disease include
A intention tremor
B 'clasp-knife' rigidity
C choreo-athetosis
D delayed relaxation of the tendon reflexes
E delayed initiation of movements

Answers
24 A C
25 A C E
26 A B D
27 A B C

28 none
29 A B C D E
30 A B C D E
31 C E

32
Tests useful in assessing the following spinal tracts include
A heel-shin test — lateral cortico-spinal tracts
B pain sensation — spino-cerebellar tracts
C joint position sensation — posterior columns
D facial pain sensation — spinal tract of the fifth cranial nerve
E pressure sensation — lateral spino-thalamic tracts

33
The lateral spino-thalamic tract of the spinal cord
A transmits pain sensation from the same side of the body
B crosses to the opposite side in the medial lemniscus
C transmits contralateral light touch sensation
D statifies fibres from the lowest spinal segments innermost
E crosses from the thalamus to the contralateral parietal lobe

34
Loss of tendon reflexes is characteristic of
A proximal myopathy
B peripheral neuropathy
C syringomyelia
D myasthenia gravis
E tabes dorsalis

35
An absent plantar response is an expected finding in
A cold feet associated with hypothermia
B spinal shock following cord transection
C paralysis of flexor hallucis longus
D L5 sensory radiculopathy
E transverse myelitis

36
The segmental innervation of the following tendon reflexes is
A biceps jerk — C5–C6
B triceps jerk — C6–C7
C supinator jerk — C5–C6
D knee jerk — L3–L4
E ankle jerk — L5–S1

37
The following statements about bladder innervation are true
A sacral cord lesions usually produce urinary retention
B thoracic cord lesions produce urinary incontinence or retention
C pelvic nerve parasympathetic stimulation causes bladder emptying
D pudendal nerve lesions produce automatic bladder emptying
E the L1–L2 segment sympathetic outflow mediates bladder relaxation

38
The following cerebrospinal fluid (CSF) findings are normal
A protein content = 0.2–0.5 g/L
B cell count = 10–20 neutrophil leucocytes per ml
C glucose = 2.2–4.5 mmol/L
D IgG content = 50% of the total CSF protein
E pressure = 200–300 mm of CSF

39
The following statements about electroencephalography are true
A the EEG shows more marked changes in chronic than acute disease
B the EEG is more often abnormal in meningiomas than gliomas
C the EEG is typically normal in petit mal epilepsy
D posterior fossa disease usually produces a characteristic EEG
E a normal EEG excludes the diagnosis of grand mal epilepsy

Answers
32 C D
33 C
34 B C E
35 A B C

36 A B C D E
37 A B C E
38 A C
39 none

40
The following statements about the Glasgow coma scale are true
A the best response to an arousal stimulus should be measured
B appropriate motor responses to verbal commands = score 6
C spontaneous eye opening = score 4
D verbal responses with normal speech and orientation = score 5
E the minimum total score = 3

41
The diagnosis of brain death is supported by
A pin-point pupils
B absent corneal reflexes
C absent vestibulo-ocular responses to caloric testing
D absence of spontaneous respiration
E preservation of the cough and gag reflexes

42
Typical features of prefrontal lobe lesions include
A positive grasp reflex
B astereognosis
C sensory dysphasia
D olfactory hallucinations
E social disinhibition

43
Typical features of posterior parietal lobe lesions include
A lower homonymous quadrantanopia
B constructional apraxia
C perceptual rivalry
D motor dysphasia
E agnosia and acalculia

44
Typical features of temporal lobe lesions of the cortex include
A visual, auditory or olfactory hallucinations
B upper homonymous quadrantanopia
C motor dysphasia
D déjà vu phenomena
E dyspraxia

45
Typical causes of papilloedema include
A migraine
B central retinal vein thrombosis
C cranial arteritis
D chronic ventilatory failure
E chronic glaucoma

46
Typical causes of oculomotor and abducent nerve palsies include
A refractive errors in childhood
B diabetes mellitus
C raised intracranial pressure
D polyarteritis nodosa
E herpes zoster

47
Jerking bidirectional nystagmus present looking in either direction
A is compatible with cerebellar hemisphere disease
B is indicative of a brainstem disorder
C is compatible with a vestibular nerve lesion
D is typically accompanied by vertigo and tinnitus
E usually ceases following closure of the eyes

Answers
40 A B C D E
41 B C D
42 A E
43 A B C E

44 A B D
45 B C D
46 B C D
47 A B

48
The characteristic features of trigeminal neuralgia include
A pain lasting several hours at a time
B pain precipitated by touching the face and/or chewing
C absence of the corneal reflex
D predominance in young females
E pain and facial spasm confined to the ophthalmic division

49
The typical features of Bell's facial nerve palsy include
A impairment of the orbicularis oculi on the affected side
B preservation of forehead wrinkling on the affected side
C ipsilateral loss of taste sensation on the posterior tongue
D rapid onset of improvement augurs a better prognosis
E loss of skin sensation on the affected side of the face

50
The typical features of Meniere's disease include
A sudden onset of vertigo, nausea and vomiting
B progressive sensorineural deafness and tinnitus
C rotatory jerking nystagmus and ataxic gait
D positional nystagmus usually persists between attacks
E restoration of hearing following effective treatment

51
Typical causes of vertigo include
A petit mal epilepsy
B acoustic neuroma
C vestibular neuronitis
D salicylate therapy
E otitis media

52
Wasting and fasciculation of the tongue is a feature of
A pseudo-bulbar palsy
B myasthenia gravis
C tertiary neurosyphilis
D nasopharyngeal carcinoma
E Paget's disease of the skull

53
Expected findings in Horner's syndrome include
A excessive facial sweating
B enophthalmos
C paralysis of accommodation
D pupillary constriction
E complete ptosis

54
Typical features of generalised epilepsy include
A loss of consciousness accompanied by symmetrical EEG discharge
B EEG focus arising in the diencephalon
C lesion demonstrable on CT brain scanning
D induction by photic stimulation
E induction by hyperventilation

55
The clinical features of tonic-clonic seizures include
A prodromal phase lasting hours or days
B onset with an audible cry due to the aura
C sustained spasm of all muscles lasting 30 seconds
D interrupted jerking movements lasting 30 seconds
E flaccid post-ictal stage of relaxation

Answers
48 B E
49 A D
50 A B C
51 B C D E

52 D E
53 B D
54 A B D E
55 A C D E

56
The typical features of absence (petit mal) seizures include
A loss of consciousness lasting 10 seconds
B onset at the age 25–30 years
C synchronous 3 per second spike and wave EEG abnormality
D hemiparesis lasting several hours post-ictally
E sleepiness lasting several hours post-ictally

57
Characteristic features of temporal lobe epilepsy include
A complex partial seizure with loss of awareness
B hallucinations of smell, taste, hearing or vision
C déjà vu phenomena associated with intense emotion
D progression to tonic-clonic seizure
E Todd's hemiparesis lasting several hours post-ictally

58
Recognised causes of epilepsy in elderly patients include
A alcohol abuse
B hypoglycaemia
C cerebrovascular disease
D Stoke-Adams attacks
E cerebral tumour

59
The following are compatible with a diagnosis of narcolepsy
A episodic limb paralysis associated with intense emotion
B transient blackouts causing recurrent falls
C terrifying hallucinations on waking or falling asleep
D sleep paralysis on waking or falling asleep
E association with HLA-DR2

60
The management of grand mal epilepsy should include
A hospital admission following episodes
B return to driving after 2 years free of day-time seizures
C irrevocable loss of an HGV driving licence
D combined primidone and phenobarbitone therapy
E phenytoin, carbamazepine or sodium valproate therapy

61
Features suggesting epilepsy as the cause of blackouts include
A impairment of vision heralding the attack
B urinary incontinence during the attack
C eye witness account of jerking movements during the attack
D attacks aborted by lying supine
E attacks confined to the sleeping hours

62
Complications of long-term anticonvulsant therapy include
A phenytoin — lymphadenopathy and gingival hypertrophy
B carbamazepine — drowsiness and ataxia
C sodium valproate — hair loss and tremor
D rickets and osteomalacia
E folic acid deficiency and megaloblastic anaemia

63
Clinical features of raised intracranial pressure include
A tachycardia and hypotension
B dizziness and lightheadedness
C headache aggravated by bending and straining
D behavioral and personality changes
E sixth, third or fourth cranial nerve palsies

Answers
56 A C
57 A B C
58 A B C D E
59 A C D E

60 B C E
61 B C E
62 A B C D E
63 B C D E

64
The following statements about primary brain tumours are true
A meningiomas are commonest in the middle aged
B gliomas are commonest in childhood
C most childhood brain tumours arise within the posterior fossa
D presentation with adult-onset partial seizures is typical
E acoustic neuromas usually present in the sixth and seventh decades

65
Papilloedema due to raised intracranial pressure typically produces
A severe visual impairment at presentation
B a central scotoma detectable on visual perimetry
C pain and tenderness in the affected eye
D retinal haemorrhages around the optic disc if rapid in onset
E unilateral optic atrophy in tumours of the anterior cranial fossa

66
Characteristic features of normal-pressure hydrocephalus include
A urinary incontinence
B dementia and ataxia
C cerebral atrophy
D partial simple epilepsy
E communicating hydrocephalus

67
Recognised features of migraine include
A family history of migraine
B onset before the age of puberty
C headache is invariably unilateral and throbbing
D premonitory symptoms include teichopsia
E hemiparaesthesiae or hemiparesis at onset

68
The visual phenomena of migraine
A seldom persist longer than 30 minutes
B usually develop 30 minutes after the onset of headache
C often include photophobia and scotomas
D are attributable to cerebral cortical arteriolar dilatation
E typically comprise loss of colour vision

69
There is a major risk of cerebral embolism associated with
A calf vein thrombosis
B atrial fibrillation
C atrial myxoma
D infective endocarditis
E acute rheumatic fever

70
Cerebral embolism is a likely cause of stroke given the following
A blood pressure = 240/130 mmHg
B retinal haemorrhages
C haemoglobin = 18 g/dL
D mitral stenosis
E history of amaurosis fugax

71
Typical causes of transient cerebral ischaemic attacks include
A carotid artery stenosis
B hypertension
C hypotension
D intracerebellar haemorrhage
E intracerebral tumour

Answers
64 A C D
65 D E
66 A B C E
67 A D E

68 A C
69 B C D
70 D E
71 A B C

72
Clinical features suggesting lacunar (minor) stroke include
A homonymous hemianopia
B motor or sensory dysphasia
C facial weakness and arm monoparesis
D isolated hemiparesis or hemianaesthesia
E history of hypertension or diabetes mellitus

73
Clinical features suggesting intracerebral haemorrhage include
A abrupt onset of severe headache followed by coma
B third cranial nerve palsy
C retinal haemorrhages and/or papilloedema
D onset of stroke on waking from sleep
E tinnitus, deafness and vertigo

74
Typical manifestations of brain stem infarction include
A pin-point pupils
B vertigo and diplopia
C sensory dysphasia
D severe headache
E bidirectional jerking nystagmus

75
Functional recovery following stroke is unlikely to be good if
A there is prolonged coma
B the stroke was haemorrhagic rather than embolic in origin
C there is severe hypertension
D there is a conjugate gaze palsy
E hemiplegia is left-sided rather than right-sided

76
Typical features of chronic subdural haematoma in adults include
A recall of a recent head injury
B urinary incontinence and ataxia
C epilepsy without previous headaches
D hemiplegia and hemianopia of sudden onset
E fluctuating confusional state

77
Typical features of superior sagittal sinus thrombosis include
A headache and papilloedema
B Jacksonian epilepsy
C flaccid paraparesis
D preexisting hypercoagulable state
E symptoms of local infection are absent

78
Typical features of cavernous sinus thrombosis include
A preexisting facial or sinus sepsis
B onset with headache and unilateral proptosis
C complete third, fourth and sixth cranial nerve palsies
D bilateral involvement rarely ensues
E sparing of the optic discs is characteristic

79
The typical features of spinal epidural abscess include
A absence of local pain or tenderness
B urinary incontinence and paraparesis
C peripheral blood leucocytosis
D normal isotope bone scan of the spine
E antibiotic and neurosurgical therapy are mandatory

Answers
72 C D E
73 A B C
74 A B D E
75 A B C D E

76 B E
77 A B C D E
78 A B C
79 B C E

80
Intracerebral abscess is a typical complication of
A infective endocarditis
B bronchiectasis
C frontal sinusitis
D otitis media
E head injury

81
The typical features of chronic intracerebral abscess include
A high fever, weight loss and peripheral blood leucocytosis
B epilepsy persisting after successful treatment of the abscess
C bradycardia and papilloedema
D headache, vomiting and confusion
E positive blood and CSF cultures

82
CSF protein concentrations > 1 g/L are typical findings in
A viral meningitis
B chronic intracerebral abscess
C Guillain-Barré syndrome
D spinal neurofibroma
E neurosyphilis

83
CSF glucose concentrations < 2.2 mmol/L are typical findings in
A poliomyelitis
B tuberculous meningitis
C carcinomatous meningitis
D intracerebral abscess
E pyogenic meningitis

84
The typical features of adult tuberculous meningitis include
A headache and vomiting
B fever associated with neck stiffness
C cranial nerve palsies associated with coma
D miliary tuberculosis is invariably present
E the CSF cell count >400 neutrophil leucocytes per ml

85
In the treatment of tuberculous meningitis
A prednisolone therapy should be given to most patients
B the condition is fatal unless anti-TB therapy is given
C all patients should be isolated
D rifampicin and isoniazid cross the blood-brain barrier poorly
E intrathecal streptomycin is the ideal therapy

86
Meningitis is a recognised complication of
A Lyme disease
B sarcoidosis
C typhus fever
D amoebiasis
E crytococcosis

87
In the treatment of adult pyogenic meningitis
A penicillin should be given intrathecally initially
B chloramphenicol should be given to penicillin-allergic patients
C antibiotic therapy should always be deferred pending CSF analysis
D i.v. fluid therapy should be instituted immediately
E the onset of a purpuric rash suggests drug allergy is likely

Answers
80 A B C D E
81 B C D
82 C D
83 B C E

84 A B C
85 A B
86 A B C D E
87 B D

88
Recognised causes of viral meningitis include
A herpes zoster
B polyomyelitis
C hepatitis A and HIV infection
D Echo and Coxsackie viruses
E measles and mumps viruses

89
Typical features of acute lymphocytic choriomeningitis include
A an arenavirus infection transmitted from mice and hamsters
B characteristically distinct from poliomyelitis and tuberculosis
C recovery is often incomplete with residual neurological deficit
D responds promptly to cytosine arabinoside
E CSF pleocytosis persists long after clinical resolution

90
Typical features of adult viral encephalitis include
A acute onset of headache and fever
B partial epilepsy and coma rapidly ensue
C decreased CSF glucose concentration
D temporal lobe EEG abnormalities suggest herpes simplex infection
E dysphasic syndromes and cranial nerve palsies

91
The characteristic features of acute poliomyelitis include
A incubation period of 7–14 days
B fever, headache and meningism
C muscle paralysis is greatest within the first week of onset
D muscle paralysis gradually recovers after a delay of 4 weeks
E when paralysis is permanent, spasticity and hyperreflexia ensue

92
Typical features of herpes zoster include
A the rash heals without scarring
B permanent dermatomal sensory impairment
C infection is confined to the posterior root ganglia
D pain is the first symptom before a rash appears
E treatment with acyclovir prevents post-herpetic neuralgia

93
Recognised sequelae of herpes zoster infection include
A corneal ulceration
B facial nerve palsy
C chicken pox outbreak
D transverse myelitis
E post-herpetic neuralgia

94
Syphilis should be excluded from the differential diagnosis of
A late-onset epilepsy
B progressive dementia
C stroke in young patients
D truncal or limb ataxia
E septic meningitis

95
The following statements about neurosyphilis are true
A CSF pleocytosis indicates active disease requiring therapy
B effective therapy renders the CSF syphilis serology negative
C parenteral procaine penicillin is the treatment of choice
D CSF syphilis serology is invariably positive in tabes dorsalis
E repeat CSF analysis is necessary following effective therapy

---

Answers
88 A B C D E
89 A E
90 A B E
91 A B C

92 B D
93 A B C D E
94 A B C D E
95 A C E

96
The clinical features of meningovascular syphilis include
A macular rash and generalised lymphadenopathy
B fever, headache, partial epilepsy and meningism
C CSF pleocytosis comprising numerous lymphocytes
D endarteritis obliterans producing cranial nerve palsies
E thrombosis of the anterior spinal artery producing paraparesis

97
Characteristic features of Argyll Robertson pupils include
A symmetrical pupillary dilatation
B reaction to accommodation
C atrophy and depigmentation of the iris
D absence of the cilio-spinal reflex
E slow progressive reaction to light

98
Typical features of tabes dorsalis include
A paroxysmal abdominal and girdle pains
B loss of pain sensation of the nose, perineum and feet
C bilateral ptosis and Argyll Robertson pupils
D urinary incontinence with absent ankle and plantar reflexes
E high stepping, stamping gait with muscle hypotonia

99
Typical features of general paralysis of the insane include
A onset within 5 years of infection
B rapidly progressive dementia
C tremor of the lips, tongue and head
D epilepsy with transient hemiplegia, hemianopia or dysphasia
E urinary incontinence as a result of sensory denervation

100
Epidemiological characteristics of multiple sclerosis include
A predominantly affects males
B assocation with HLA-A3, B7 and Dw2/DRw2
C affects 1 in 2000 of the UK population
D more prevalent in the tropics than in temperate climates
E lesions within the CNS are confined to the grey matter

101
The typical features of multiple sclerosis include
A invariable progression with relapses and remission
B onset often occurs before the age of puberty
C choreoathetosis and parkinsonism
D urinary urgency, frequency and incontinence
E epilepsy, dysphasia or hemiplegia

102
Recognised clinical presentations of multiple sclerosis include
A trigeminal neuralgia and atypical facial pain
B vertigo, diplopia and ataxia
C transverse myelitis and Brown-Sequard syndrome
D internuclear ophthalmoplegia with dysconjugate nystagmus
E retrobulbar neuritis and Lhermitte's (barber's chair) sign

103
Useful investigations in diagnosing multiple sclerosis include
A visual and somatosensory evoked potentials
B CT and magnetic resonance brain scanning
C CSF analysis for oligoclonal IgG bands
D electroencephalography
E electromyography

Answers
96 A B C D E
97 B C D
98 A B C D E
99 C D

100 B C
101 D
102 A B C D E
103 A B C

104
The typical features of parkinsonism include
A hypokinesia
B dementia
C intention tremor
D lead-pipe rigidity
E impaired upward gaze

105
Findings inconsistent with idiopathic Parkinson's disease include
A unilateral onset of the disorder
B emotional lability
C oculogyric crises
D extensor plantar responses
E impaired pupillary accommodation reflexes

106
The typical features of extrapyramidal movements include
A stereotyped movements in chorea
B slow imprecise movements in parkinsonism
C flinging movements in ballismus
D writhing movements in athetosis
E unpredictable movements in tics

107
Parkinsonism is a typical feature of
A post-encephalitis lethargica
B phenothiazine and butyrophenone therapy
C Wilson's disease
D repetitive head injury e.g boxing
E Alzheimer's dementia

108
Recognised features of Wilson's disease include
A autosomal recessive inheritance
B clinical onset in the neonatal period
C dementia, choreoathetosis and parkinsonism
D acute haemolytic anaemia
E increased serum caeruloplasmin concentration

109
The typical features of kernicterus include
A severe neonatal unconjugated hyperbilirubinaemia
B convulsions and opisthotonos
C mental subnormality and nerve deafness
D spastic paralysis and choreoathetosis
E complete recovery following exchange transfusion

110
The characteristic features of Huntington's chorea include
A autosomal recessive inheritance
B clinical onset before the age of puberty
C progress of dementia arrested with tetrabenazine therapy
D choreiform movements of the face and arms particularly
E cardiomyopathic changes on echocardiography

111
The clinical features of motor neurone disease include
A insidious onset in elderly males
B progressive distal muscular atrophy
C progressive bulbar palsy
D upper motor neurone signs in the lower limbs
E lower motor neurone signs in the upper limbs

Answers
104 A D E
105 B C D
106 B C D
107 A B C D E

108 A C D
109 A B C D
110 D
111 A B C D E

112
The differential diagnosis in motor neurone disease includes
A syringomyelia
B diabetic amyotrophy
C cervical myelopathy
D paraneoplastic syndrome
E meningovascular syphilis

113
Typical features of cervical radiculopathy include
A pathognomonic X-ray abnormalities of the cervical spine
B radicular pain in the arm and shoulder
C painful limitation of movements of the cervical spine
D C8-T1 sensory and/or motor loss in the upper limb
E neurosurgical intervention is often required

114
Typical features of the lumbago-sciatica syndrome include
A increased lumbar lordosis apparent radiologically
B aggravation of the pain on coughing and sneezing
C tenderness on pressure over the greater sciatic notch
D loss of both the ankle and knee tendon jerks
E wasting of the calf muscles or the presence of a foot drop

115
The clinical features suggesting an extramedullary rather than intramedullary cord lesion include
A early onset of anal/bladder sphincter impairment
B dissociate sensory loss in the lower limbs
C late onset of radicular symptoms or signs
D lower limb hyperreflexia and extensor plantar responses
E preservation of sensation in the sacral dermatomes

116
The following statements about spinal cord compression are true
A metastatic disease is a more common cause than primary tumour
B the CSF protein concentration is likely to be normal
C local spinal pain and tenderness usually precedes motor weakness
D urinary urgency is commonly the presenting feature
E myelography is best undertaken following neurosurgical referral

117
Recognised causes of paraplegia include
A intracranial parasagittal meningioma
B vitamin B_{12} deficiency
C tuberculosis of the thoracic spine
D anterior spinal artery thrombosis
E spinal neurofibromas and gliomas

Answers
112 A B C D E
113 B D
114 B C E

115 none
116 A C E
117 A B C D E

118
The clinical features of the Brown-Sequard syndrome include
A pain and temperature sensory loss in the contralateral leg
B proprioceptive sensory loss in the ipsilateral leg
C an extensor plantar response in the ipsilateral leg
D hyperreflexia and weakness of the contralateral leg
E hyperaesthetic dermatome on the opposite side of the lesion

119
In the treatment of established paraplegia
A prophylactic antibiotics are indicated to prevent urinary sepsis
B pressure sores are not likely to occur unless sensation is lost
C urinary retention usually requires long-term catheterisation
D flexor spasms and contractures are unavoidable despite therapy
E constipation requires dietary treatment and regular enemas

120
Characteristic features of Friedreich's ataxia include
A posterior column, spinocerebellar and corticospinal tract atrophy
B spinal scoliosis, pes cavus and truncal ataxia
C absent ankle jerks and extensor plantar responses
D jerking bidirectional nystagmus and dysarthria
E hypertrophic cardiomyopathy and diabetes mellitus

121
Recognised features of peroneal muscular atrophy include
A wasting of the distal limb muscles and bilateral foot drop
B loss of the tendon and plantar reflexes
C Argyll Robertson pupils and optic atrophy
D progression of muscle wasting above the knees and elbows
E mental subnormality and multiple cranial neuropathies

122
The typical features of syringomyelia include
A slow insidious progression of the disease
B dissociate sensory loss with normal touch and position sense
C loss of one or more upper limb tendon reflexes is invariable
D wasting of the small muscles of the hands
E hyperreflexia of the lower limbs and extensor plantar responses

123
Disorganised (Charcot's) joints are a recognised feature of
A tabes dorsalis
B syringomyelia
C motor neurone disease
D diabetic neuropathy
E amyotrophic lateral sclerosis

124
Recognised features of neurofibromatosis include
A autosomal dominant trait transmitted on chromosome 17
B cafe-au-lait spots and axillary skin freckling
C association with multiple endocrine neoplasias
D intraspinal and intracranial neuromas and meningiomas
E pigmented iris hamartomas (Lisch nodules)

Answers
118 A B C
119 A E
120 A B C D E

121 A B C
122 A B C D E
123 A B D
124 A B C D E

125
Recognised features of severe vitamin B$_{12}$ deficiency include
A mononeuritis multiplex
B optic atrophy
C confusion and dementia
D spastic paraparesis
E sensory ataxia

126
Recognised features of Wernicke's encephalopathy include
A profound nicotinamide deficiency
B conjugate gaze palsy and jerking nystagmus
C association with anorexia nervosa and alcoholism
D loss of the pupillary reflexes
E reversible short-term memory loss and dementia

127
Typical features of the carpal tunnel syndrome include
A remission during pregnancy
B wasting of the dorsal interossei and lumbricals
C invariably unilateral if producing night waking
D association with acromegaly and hypothyroidism
E complication of both rheumatoid arthritis and amyloidosis

128
Recognised causes of mononeuritis multiplex include
A rheumatoid arthritis
B sarcoidosis
C polyarteritis nodosa
D diabetes mellitus
E systemic lupus erythematosus

129
Typical features of neuralgic amyotrophy include
A onset following immunisation or infection
B severe pain and motor impairment in the spinal segments C5–C6
C profound sensory loss in the dermatomes C8–T1
D prompt response to corticosteroid therapy
E recovery from paralysis usually takes several months

130
Recognised causes of a generalised polyneuropathy include
A bronchial carcinoma and lymphoproliferative disorders
B rheumatoid arthritis and systemic lupus erythematosus
C folate, B$_{12}$, B$_1$, B$_2$, B$_6$ and E vitamin deficiencies
D drugs especially cotrimoxazole, phenytoin and mianserin
E diabetes mellitus and chronic renal failure

131
Clinical features typical of the following polyneuropathies include
A predominantly motor loss — lead poisoning
B predominantly sensory loss — post-inflammatory polyneuropathy
C painful sensory impairment — alcohol abuse
D sparing of the cranial nerves — sarcoidosis
E prominent postural hypotension — diabetes mellitus

Answers
125 B CD E
126 B CD
127 D E
128 A BCDE

129 A BE
130 A BCDE
131 A CE

132
The presence of the following is likely to be useful in the identification of the cause of a polyneuropathy
A peripheral blood punctate basophilia
B atrophic glossitis and weight loss
C hyponatraemia with urinary osmolality = 300 mOsmol/kg
D recent discovery of Kayser-Fleischer corneal rings
E family history of neurofibromatosis

133
The typical features of Guillain-Barré polyneuropathy include
A onset within 4 weeks of an acute infective illness
B severe back pain and peripheral paraesthesiae
C ascending flaccid paralysis with areflexia
D sparing of the respiratory and facial nerves
E normal CSF protein concentration and cell count

134
Non-metastatic neurological complications of malignancy include
A meralgia paraesthetica
B carpal tunnel syndrome
C cerebellar ataxia
D progressive dementia
E myasthenic syndrome

135
Characteristic features of myasthenia gravis include
A association with HLA-B8 and DRw3
B circulating anti-acetylcholine receptor antibodies
C onset of the disease between the ages 15–50 years
D abnormal muscle fatiguability on electromyography
E intermittent diplopia and ptosis

136
In the treatment of myasthenia gravis
A pupillary miosis, salivation and sweating typify excessive therapy
B pyridostigmine is best given with propantheline 4–8 hourly
C thymectomy is mandatory as soon as the diagnosis is confirmed
D corticosteroid therapy produces a transient myasthenic crisis
E the prognosis is significantly worse if associated with thymoma

137
The typical inheritance of the following muscular dystrophies is as shown below
A facio-scapulo-humeral type — autosomal recessive
B limb-girdle type — autosomal dominant
C Duchenne type — X-linked recessive
D ocular type — autosomal dominant
E dystrophia myotonica — autosomal dominant

138
The typical features of Duchenne muscular dystrophy include
A presentation in the third year of life
B calf muscle hypertrophy
C difficulty in rising from the floor
D normal serum creatine phosphokinase concentration
E death is usually due to cardiac and respiratory failure

139
The typical features of dystrophia myotonica include
A onset with a proximal myopathy in the first and second decades
B diabetes mellitus, frontal baldness and gonadal atrophy
C ptosis and wasting of the facial and sternomastoid muscles
D cataracts, dysphagia and cardiomyopathy
E survival is rare beyond the age of 40 years

Answers
132 A B
133 A B C
134 C D E
135 A B C D E

136 A C D E
137 C D E
138 A B C E
139 B C D

140
Recognised causes of proximal myopathy include
A hypothyroidism and hyperthyroidism
B type I diabetes mellitus
C Cushing's syndrome and acromegaly
D Addisonian pernicious anaemia
E chronic alcohol abuse

Answers
140 A C E

Dermatology

1
The following statements about the skin are true
A the weight of an adult's skin is approximately 4 kg
B the surface area of an adult is approximately two metres^2
C keratinocytes comprise one third of epidermal cell numbers
D Langerhan cells synthesise vitamin D in the epidermis
E eccrine sweat glands account for specific skin and body odours

2
In the terminology of skin lesions
A papules are solid skin elevations > 2 cm in diameter
B nodules are solid skin masses > 0.5 cm in diameter
C vesicles are fluid-containing skin elevations > 0.5 cm in diameter
D petechiae are pinhead-sized macules of blood within the skin
E macules are small raised areas of skin of altered colour

3
Properties of vehicles for topical skin treatments include
A creams comprise grease to moisturise dry skin
B ointments comprise water, grease and an emulsifier
C pastes comprise grease and an alcohol
D shake lotions comprise water and powder to aid skin cooling
E lotions comprise water or alcohol for use in hairy areas

4
Effects of topical corticosteroid therapy include
A dermal atrophy most marked in the face and body folds
B striae in the body folds particularly
C absence of hypothalamo-pituitary-adrenal axis suppression
D decreased hair growth particularly of the beard
E spread of skin infection

5
Characteristic features of eczema include
A epidermal oedema (spongiosis) and intra-epidermal vesicles
B delayed hypersensitivity reaction in seborrhoeic eczema
C increased serum IgA concentration in discoid (nummular) eczema
D eyelid oedema in allergic contact eczema
E persistence of childhood atopic eczema into adulthood

6
Typical sensitising agents in contact eczema include
A aluminium
B colophony
C lanolin
D rubber
E ethanol

Answers
1 A B
2 B D
3 D E

4 A B E
5 A D
6 B C D

7
Typical features of psoriasis include
A well-defined erythematous plaques with adherent silvery scales
B epidermal thickening and nucleated horny layer cells (parakeratosis)
C induction of plaques by local trauma (Koebner phenomenon)
D an association with HLA-CW6
E exacerbation by propranolol and lithium carbonate therapy

8
The characteristic clinical features of psoriasis include
A sparing of the skin over the head, face and neck
B guttate psoriasis predominantly affecting the elderly
C nail changes with pitting and onycholysis
D oligoarthritis in 5% particularly associated with nail changes
E red non-scaly skin areas in the natal cleft and submammary folds

9
Appropriate therapeutic schedules in psoriasis include
A dithranol cream for facial plaques
B calcipotriol ointment for flexural plaques
C tar-steroid combinations during withdrawal of steroid creams
D medium wave UVA exposure from sunbeds
E combined psoralen-UVA photochemotherapy and isotretinoin

10
The typical features of acne vulgaris include
A involvement of pilosebaceous glands and their ducts
B distribution over the face and upper torso
C infection with the skin commensal *Propionibacterium acnes*
D increased sebum production containing excess free fatty acids
E open and closed comedones, inflammatory papules, nodules and cysts

11
Recognised agents inducing acneiform eruptions include
A tars and chlorinated hydrocarbons
B androgenic steroids and corticosteroids
C oral contraceptives
D lithium carbonate
E anticonvulsants

12
Therapies of proven value in acne vulgaris include
A oral antibiotic therapy e.g. oxytetracycline and erythromycin
B topical preparations of benzoyl peroxide and retinoic acid
C low dose oral oestrogen therapy
D anti-androgen therapy e.g. cyproterone acetate
E oral isotretinoin to reduce sebum secretion

13
The characteristic features of rosacea include
A predominantly affects adolescents
B increased secretion of sebum with comedones
C facial erythema, telangiectasia, pustules and papules
D rhinophyma, conjunctivitis and keratitis
E absent response to oral oxytetracycline therapy

Answers

7 A B C D E
8 C D E
9 B C E

10 A B C D E
11 A B C D E
12 A B D E
13 C D

14
The typical features of lichen planus include
A involvement of the skin, nails, hair and mucous membranes
B dense subepidermal lymphocytic infiltration on histology
C itchy, purplish, polygonal, shiny skin papules
D hypopigmention of the sites of old lesions
E complete resolution following topical steroid therapy

15
Characteristic features in Henoch-Schonlein vasculitis include
A palpable purpuric rash particularly over the buttocks
B lymphocytic infiltration of capillary endothethelium
C leucocytoclastic vasculitis and endothelial IgA deposition
D polyarthritis and mononeuritis multiplex
E corticosteroid therapy is mandatory

16
Systemic causes of pruritus include
A oral contraceptives and pregnancy
B hypothyroidism and hyperthyroidism
C lymphoproliferative and myeloproliferative diseases
D iron deficiency anaemia
E opiate and antidepressant drug therapy

17
Skin diseases associated with marked pruritus include
A cutaneous vasculitis
B lichen planus
C atopic eczema
D seborrhoeic keratosis
E dermatitis herpetiformis

18
Skin diseases associated with blistering eruptions include
A erythema multiforme
B dermatitis herpetiformis
C pemphigoid
D pemphigus vulgaris
E guttate psoriasis

19
Skin diseases associated with HIV infection include
A seborrhoeic eczema
B oral candidiasis
C oral hairy leukoplakia
D lichen planus
E Kaposi's sarcoma

20
Skin diseases associated with photosensitivity include
A variegate and hepatic porphyrias
B atopic eczema
C drug reactions to phenothiazine, thiazide and tetracycline
D pyoderma gangrenosum
E pityriasis rosea

21
The typical features of erythema multiforme include
A target-like skin lesions of the hands, and distal limbs
B skin eruption lasting 6–12 weeks
C absence of vesiculation or blistering
D involvement of the eyes, genitalia and mouth
E association with underlying systemic malignancy

Answers
14 A B C
15 A C
16 A B C D E
17 B C E

18 A B C D
19 A B C E
20 A B C
21 A D

22
Recognised causes of erythema multiforme include
A herpes simplex infection
B mycoplasmal pneumonia
C sulphonamide therapy
D systemic lupus erythematosus
E pregnancy and oral contraceptives

23
The typical features of erythema nodosum include
A red hot tender nodules over the shins
B lesions disappear over 1–2 weeks
C fever, malaise and polyarthralgia
D oral and genital mucosal ulceration
E predominantly affects the elderly

24
Recognised causes of erythema nodosum include
A sarcoidosis
B beta-haemolytic streptococcal infection
C inflammatory bowel disease
D tuberculosis
E sulphonamide and contraceptive drug therapy

25
Cutaneous manifestations of systemic malignancy include
A generalised pruritus
B acanthosis nigricans
C late-onset dermatomyositis
D generalised hyperpigmentation
E seborrhoeic eczema

26
Typical features of melanocytic naevi include
A usualy present from birth
B development after the age of 40 years
C junctional naevi are smooth, papillomatous, hairy nodules
D intradermal naevi are circular, brown macules < 1 cm in diameter
E 1% life-time risk of malignant transformation

27
Typical features of malignant melanoma include
A changing appearance of a preceding melanocytic naevus
B diameter of the lesion > 0.5 cm
C irregular colour, border and elevation
D personal or family history of melanoma
E painless, expanding, subungual area of pigmentation

28
The typical features of seborrhoeic keratosis include
A appearance before the age of 30 years
B discrete irregular lesions in light-exposed skin areas
C yellow-brown, pedunculated lesions on the trunk or face
D lesion exhibits greasy scaling and tiny keratin plugs
E eventual transition to squamous cell carcinoma

29
The typical features of basal cell carcinoma include
A predominantly affects the elderly
B metastatic spread to the lungs if untreated
C occurrence in areas exposed to light or X-irradiation
D papule with surface telangiectasia or ulcerated nodule
E unresponsive to radiotherapy

Answers
22 A B C D E
23 A C
24 A B C D E
25 A B C D

26 none
27 A B C D E
28 C D
29 A C D

30
The typical features of squamous cell carcinoma include
A occurrence in areas exposed to light or X-irradiation
B arise from malignant transformation of the Langerhan cells
C preceded by leukoplakia on the lips, mouth or genitalia
D metastatic spread to the liver and lungs
E unresponsive to radiotherapy

Answers
30 A C

Psychiatry

1

Prevalence rates of psychiatric illness in the UK include

A 5% of the general adult population

B 30% of patients attending their general practitioner

C 30% of patients attending hospital medical outpatient clinics

D 30% of patients admitted to general medical wards

E schizophrenia in 5% of the population

2

Aetiological factors in psychiatric illness include

A family history of psychiatric illness

B parental loss or dysharmony in childhood

C stressful life events and difficulties

D chronic physical ill-health

E social isolation

3

Important factors in the assessment of mental state include

A general appearance, behaviour and speech

B mood state and thought content

C abnormal beliefs and delusions

D abnormal perceptions and hallucinations

E intellect and cognitive function

4

Intellectual impairment should be suspected in the presence of

A incoherent thought processes

B impaired long-term memory

C inappropriate optimism and elation

D disorientation in time and place

E impaired serial 7s test and arithmetic ability

5

The following psychiatric definitions are true

A delusions — unreasonably persistent, firmly held false beliefs

B illusions — abnormal perceptions of normal external stimuli

C hallucinations — abnormal perceptions without external stimuli

D depersonalisation — perception of altered reality

E phobia — abnormal fear leading to avoidance behaviour

6

Cardinal elements in behavioural therapy include

A self-awareness of maladaptive patterns of learned behaviour

B systematic desensitisation and flooding

C operant conditioning and reinforcement

D exploration of repressed unpleasant experiences

E modification of negative patterns of thinking

7

Cardinal elements in cognitive therapy include

A restructuring psychological conflicts and behaviour

B identification of negative patterns of automatic thoughts

C awareness of connections between thoughts, mood and behaviour

D reorientation of negative views of the past, present and future

E personality assessment and transactional analysis

Answers

1 B C D

2 A B C D E

3 A B C D E

4 D E

5 A B C D E

6 B C

7 B C D

8
Typical features of acute confusional states include
A impaired consciousness particularly in the evening
B impaired attention, concentration and speed of thought
C impaired memory, registration, recall and retention
D illusions, hallucinations and delusions
E anxiety, irritability and depression

9
Typical features of dementia include
A loss of intellectual function without impaired consciousness
B impairment of judgement, abstract thought and problem-solving
C impairment of long-term memory without loss of short-term memory
D personality change with disinhibition and loss of social awareness
E psychomotor retardation, anxiety and depression

10
Typical features of schizophrenia include
A thought insertion and thought broadcasting
B delusions and passivity feelings
C visual hallucinations
D thought disorder and thought block
E poverty of speech, social withdrawal and flat affect

11
Features indicating a good prognosis in schizophrenia include
A abrupt onset of symptoms
B absence of affective symptoms
C schizoid personality
D catatonic symptoms
E family history of schizophrenia

12
The typical features of depression include
A depressed mood for most of the day
B insomnia or hypersomnia
C loss of pleasure, self-esteem and hope
D loss of energy, libido and interest
E psychomotor retardation and suicidal thoughts

13
The typical features of mania include
A high self-confidence and self-esteem
B reduction in sleep and food intake
C flight of ideas and rhyming speech
D grandiose delusions and reckless behaviour
E impaired attention and concentration

14
Clinical features of generalised anxiety disorders include
A feelings of worthlessness and excessive guilt
B depersonalisation and derealisation
C feelings of apprehension and impending disaster
D breathlessness, dizziness, sweating and palpitation
E claustrophobia and agoraphobia

15
Diseases mimicking anxiety disorders include
A alcohol withdrawal
B hyperthyroidism
C hypoglycaemia
D temporal lobe epilepsy
E phaeochromocytoma

Answers
 8 A B C D E
 9 A B D E
10 A B D E
11 A D

12 A B C D E
13 A B C D E
14 B C D
15 A B C D E

16
Typical features of panic disorder include
A loss of libido, anhedonia and irritability
B recurrent unpredictable attacks of intense anxiety
C chest pain, palpitation and breathlessness
D delusions and auditory hallucinations
E association with primary affective disorders

17
Typical features of phobic disorder include
A predominance in young males
B history of specific childhood trauma
C avoidance of public transport and shopping areas
D sudden intense attacks of breathlessness and faintness
E good response to benzodiazepine therapy

18
Typical features of obsessive compulsive disorder include
A consciously-resisted unwanted thoughts and impulses
B conscientiousness with perfectionistic personality
C short-lived disability without relapses
D association with schizophrenia and depression
E response to clomipramine and behaviour therapy

19
Typical features of hysterical disorder include
A conscious attempt to manipulate and/or malinger
B previous history of multiple recurrent somatic complaints
C co-existent neurological disease
D gait disturbance or sensory or motor disorder in the limbs
E pseudoseizures, blindness or aphonia

20
Typical features of anorexia nervosa include
A only adolescent girls are affected
B duration of amenorrhoea > 3 months
C weight loss > 25% or weight < 25% below normal
D normal perception of body weight and image
E retardation of physical sexual development

21
Typical features of bulimia nervosa include
A age of onset at puberty
B dramatic weight loss
C lack of control of binge-eating
D self-induced vomiting and purgation
E hospital admission required to control the disorder

22
Criteria for the diagnosis of alcohol dependence include
A increasing tolerance of the effects of alcohol
B repeated withdrawal symptoms
C priority of drinking over other activities
D progression to drinking spirits
E relief of withdrawal symptoms by further drinking

23
Alcohol abuse should be suspected in patients presenting with
A painless diarrhoea and/or vomiting
B atrial fibrillation and/or hypertension
C weight gain and/or gout
D peripheral neuropathy and/or epilepsy
E weight gain and/or insomnia

Answers
16 B C E
17 C D
18 A B D E
19 B C D E

20 B C
21 C D
22 B C E
23 A B C D E

24
The typical features of alcohol withdrawal include
A early-morning waking with anxiety and tremor
B visual or auditory hallucinations
C amnesia and epileptic seizures
D depression and morbid jealousy
E ataxia, nystagmus and ophthalmoplegia

25
Recognised features of benzodiazepine withdrawal include
A heightened sensory perception
B hallucinations and delusions
C epilepsy and ataxia
D manic-depressive-like disorder
E poverty of ideas and speech

26
Risk factors for suicide following attempted suicide include
A female sex and age < 45 years
B self-poisoning rather than more violent methods of self-harm
C absence of either a suicide note or previous suicide attempts
D chronic physical or psychiatric illness
E living alone and/or recently separated from partner

27
Indications for ECT in depressive illness include
A severe depression with paranoid delusions
B depressive stupor producing nutritional difficulties
C major risk of suicide requiring rapid therapeutic response
D unresponsive to or intolerant of oral antidepressant therapy
E depression associated with panic disorder

Answers
24 A B C
25 A B C

26 D E
27 A B C D

Clinical Pharmacology and toxicology

1
The following statements about drug metabolism are true
A maximum apparent volume of distribution = volume of total body water

B first order elimination = rate of renal clearance of a drug

C drug clearance = amount of the drug removed from plasma per hour

D first-pass elimination = degree of drug excretion in the first hour

E bioavailability = amount of the drug bound to specific receptors

2
The following statements about pharmacokinetics are true
A 50% of steady state concentration is achieved in one half-life

B the drug half-life = time taken to eliminate half the dose given

C steady state is achieved after approximately 5 half-lives

D drug bioavailability is enhanced by intravenous administration

E drug absorption and excretion are reduced in non-ionised states

3
The following statements about drug absorption are true
A oral drug absorption is reduced if nausea or pain are present

B 7–10% of drugs given by pressurised aerosols reach the lungs

C buccal and transdermal routes avoid first-pass hepatic metabolism

D rectal administration avoids presystemic hepatic elimination

E drug absorption within the stomach is enhanced by food or alcohol

4
The following examples of pharmacokinetic variability are true
A lipid-soluble drug bioavailability is enhanced by food

B chronic liver disease reduces the bioavailability of propranolol

C hypoalbuminaemia decreases drug concentrations in the free form

D impaired neonatal glucuronidation increases chloramphenicol toxicity

E ampicillin increases plasma concentrations of oral contraceptives

---

Answers
1 none
2 A C

3 A B C
4 A D

181

5
The following specific receptor types are occupied by agonists and antagonists listed below
A $alpha_1$ adrenergic — noradrenaline — prazosin
B $alpha_2$ adrenergic — noradrenaline — yohimbine
C $beta_1$ adrenergic — adrenaline — atenolol
D muscarinic cholinergic — acetylcholine — atropine
E H_2 histaminergic — histamine — cimetidine

6
The following statements about adverse drug reactions are true
A type B reactions are dose-dependent and less common than type A
B type A reactions are idiosyncratic and non-dose-dependent
C type B reactions have higher morbidity/mortality rates than type A
D type B reactions are often related to allergic mechanisms
E type A reactions usually result from aberrant metabolic pathways

7
Drugs inducing hepatic enzymatic drug metabolism include
A rifampicin
B carbamazepine
C phenytoin
D cotrimoxazole
E metronidazole

8
Drugs inhibiting hepatic enzymatic drug metabolism include
A allopurinol
B cimetidine
C cotrimoxazole
D amiodarone
E erythromycin

9
Examples of pharmacodynamic interactions include
A opiates and benzodiazepines producing synergism
B diazepam and flumazenil — receptor agonist/antagonist
C bromocriptine and metoclopramide — dopaminergic agonist/antagonist
D chlorpromazine and chlorpheniramine — cholinergic antagonists
E dobutamine and atenolol — $beta_1$ adrenergic agonist/antagonist

10
Examples of pharmacokinetic interactions include
A allopurinol inhibits the metabolism of azathioprine
B propantheline delays gastric emptying and the absorption of drugs
C digoxin and verapamil compete for renal tubular secretion
D cholestyramine binds many drugs and impairs drug absorption
E antibiotics alter gut flora disrupting enterohepatic drug cycling

11
The following statements about self-poisoning are true
A the majority of patients are middle-aged and/or suicidal
B 50% of episodes are associated with alcohol intoxication
C 66% of patients ingest drugs prescribed for family members
D 50% of patients have a previous history of self-poisoning
E 75% of patients repeat self-poisoning within 12 months

Answers
  5 A B C D E
  6 D
  7 A B C
  8 A B C D E

  9 A B C D E
10 A B C D E
11 B C D

12
Clinical features suggestive of self-poisoning include
A coma in patients under the age of 40 years
B strabismus and nystagmus in young patients
C evidence of self-injury e.g. scars on the forearms
D evidence of needle tracks suggesting i.v. drug abuse
E circumoral acneiform rash suggesting solvent abuse

13
Immediate measures in the management of self-poisoning include
A identification of the ingested poison
B use of specific antidotes and antagonists
C maintenance of the airway and respiratory function
D maintenance of blood pressure and circulatory function
E induction of vomiting by salt water

14
The following statements about gastric lavage are true
A lavage is preferable to the use of ipecacuanha in children
B the position of the tube should be checked under X-ray control
C in comatose patients, endotracheal intubation must precede lavage
D patients should lie on their left side in a head-down tilt
E activated charcoal should be given following completion of lavage

15
The use of gastric lavage or ipecacuanha following self-poisoning
A should be avoided if petrolleum distillates have been ingested
B with aspirin is unlikely to be helpful 8 hours after ingestion
C with tricyclic antidepressants is indicated 8 hours post-ingestion
D should always be undertaken if paraquat has been ingested
E should never be undertaken in hypothermic patients

16
Haemodialysis usefully enhances the elimination of
A phenobarbitone
B methanol
C ethylene glycol
D lithium carbonate
E salicylates

17
Haemoperfusion usefully enhances the elimination of
A carbamazepine
B paracetamol
C phenelzine
D theophylline
E amitriptyline

18
Typical features 12 hours after paracetamol poisoning include
A nausea, vomiting and abdominal pain
B coma and internuclear ophthalmoplegia
C prolongation of the prothrombin time
D metabolic acidosis and hypoglycaemia
E prevention of liver damage with methionine

Answers
12 A B C D E
13 C D
14 C D E

15 A C D
16 A B C D E
17 A D
18 A E

19
Typical features 8 hours after salicylate poisoning include
A coma and dilated pupils in adults
B deafness, tinnitus and blurred vision
C hypokalaemia and respiratory alkalosis in adults
D hyperventilation, sweating and restlessness
E an empty stomach before gastric lavage

20
Typical features following benzodiazepine poisoning include
A ataxia, dysarthria, nystagmus and drowsiness
B systemic hypotension and respiratory depression
C nausea, vomiting and diarrhoea
D convulsions, muscle spasms and papilloedema
E dramatic response to flumazenil therapy

21
Typical features following barbiturate poisoning include
A hypotension and hypothermia
B coma and respiratory depression
C skin blisters on dependent areas
D sweating, restlessness and hallucinations
E nausea, vomiting and abdominal pain

22
Typical features following amitriptyline poisoning include
A coma, hyperreflexia and extensor plantar responses
B warm, dry skin and dry mouth
C dilated pupils and internuclear ophthalmoplegia
D hallucinations and urinary retention
E convulsions and cardiac tachyarrhythmias

23
Poisoning with drugs containing dextropropoxyphene produces
A hyperventilation and agitation
B coma with pin-point pupils and hypotonia
C hypotension and respiratory depression
D high plasma paracetamol concentration
E absence of a response to naloxone therapy

24
Typical features of morphine poisoning include
A nausea, vomiting and pallor
B coma, miotic pupils and hyporeflexia
C hypoventilation and hypothermia
D hypotension and respiratory arrest
E non-cardiac pulmonary oedema

25
Typical features of elemental iron poisoning include
A nausea, vomiting and abdominal pain
B tachypnoea and tachycardia
C acute gastrointestinal haemorrhage
D encephalopathy and circulatory failure
E acute renal and hepatic failure

26
Typical features of lithium carbonate poisoning include
A nausea, vomiting and diarrhoea
B thirst and polyuria
C ataxia, dysarthria and coma
D hypernatraemia and hypokalaemia
E prolongation of the QRS and QT intervals and AV block on ECG

Answers
19 B C D
20 A E
21 A B C
22 A B C D E

23 B C D
24 A B C D E
25 A B C D E
26 A B C D E

27
Findings consistent with ethanol poisoning include
A drowsiness, dysarthria, ataxia and nystagmus
B hyponatraemia and hypoglycaemia
C hypernatraemia and hypothermia
D hyperventilation and metabolic acidosis
E coma and convulsions

28
Methanol poisoning characteristically produces
A the features of ethanol intoxication
B abdominal pain, vomiting and convulsions
C fixed dilated pupils and papilloedema
D severe metabolic acidosis due to lactic acid
E optic atrophy and permanent blindness

29
Ethylene glycol poisoning typically produces
A coma and convulsions
B papilloedema and ophthalmoplegia
C lactic acidosis and renal failure
D hypokalaemia and hypercalcaemia
E permanent blindness due to optic atrophy

30
Organophosphate poisoning is characteristically associated with
A sewage workers
B vomiting, abdominal pain and diarrhoea
C sweating, hypersalivation and bronchorrhoea
D coma, convulsions and muscle twitching
E clinical response to pyridostigmine therapy

Answers
27 A B C D E
28 B C D E

29 A B C E
30 B C D